THE PRACTICE OF CLINICAL RESEARCH

The Single Case Method

John H. Behling, Ph.D.
Esther S. Merves, M.A.

The Ohio State University

UNIVERSITY
PRESS OF
AMERICA

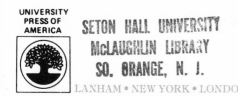

LANHAM • NEW YORK • LONDON

Copyright © 1984 by

University Press of America,™ Inc.

4720 Boston Way
Lanham, MD 20706

3 Henrietta Street
London WC2E 8LU England

ISBN (Perfect): 0-8191-4184-4
ISBN   (Cloth): 0-8191-4183-6

All University Press of America books are produced on acid-free
paper which exceeds the minimum standards set by the National
Historical Publications and Records Commission.

TABLE OF CONTENTS

PREFACE

This material has been written for the beginner. It is an illustrated discussion of single case research and is intended to focus on the methodology of single case designs. Single case methodology is sometimes referred to as N=1 studies. They were once fairly common among those doing therapy and treatment among the emotionally ill housed in mental hospitals. Discussion of these early uses of single case research will be discussed in due course. This primer of lecture notes has been divided into nine chapters. They are: (1) Introduction, (2) Research Designs, (3) Problem Definition, (4) Measurement and Instrumentation, (5) Data Collection and Processing, (6) Methods of Data Analysis, (7) Statistical Techniques, (8) Computer Application, and (9) A Final Comment.

These materials appear as notes and illustrations. The references to other researchers, thinkers, and writers are generously scattered throughout the material. Students are encouraged to read more extensively from these references. It is hoped that this primer will give the reader a new tool for not only helping her clients but improving her practice skills on the way to helping clients resolve difficulties. Yet, and perhaps more importantly, practitioners and lay persons alike may find these techniques, and this method in general, a way of controlling life and improving its quality to the satisfaction of the user. This at least has been the experience of the writers.

Esther S. Merves
John H. Behling

April, 1984

CHAPTER I

THE SINGLE CASE METHOD

Introduction

Extreme desire, intent, and commitment to any helping or human service profession does not insure effective nor efficient practice. Special training from one school or specializing in one particular mode of therapy, no matter how well known, still leaves unanswered the question of effectiveness and its documentation. However, that question has not been neglected. The abundance of recent literature on the applicability and feasibility of single case methodology for practitioners is evidenced by such texts as Evaluating Practice (Bloom and Fisher, 1982) and Empirical Clinical Practice (Jayaratne and Levy, 1979).

This methodology is simultaneously both simple and complex. Its simplicity lies in its relation to the natural experimenting we do in our everyday lives. For example, if we suspect that a certain food is causing heartburn we may avoid that food for awhile to see if that food was indeed responsible for the indigestion. Or our family physician may prescribe medication for a period of time because he thinks that the medicine will affect the ailment. The adding or withholding of food, often used in behavioral medication or token economies is a simple example of a single case methodology. Because single case designs are independent from any theoretical approach, and can be used in virtually all practice settings, with one or many clients or systems, its complexity is as a sophisticated and powerful heuristic device with which the practitioners can more fully document their practice, evaluate the success of a treatment strategy, and oftentimes involve the client as a more active participant in the therapeutic process.

The growing demand for accountability is heightened in the human services. Good work, training, and intent do not satisfy the requirements of accountability. Documentation of effective services must go beyond knowing how many clients were served in a fiscal year. Program goals are necessary but their formulation does not answer pertinent questions such as: Has the service had any effect on client functioning? Has counseling reduced distress? And finally, did the client change because of the treatment?

1

Our accountability does not come in a lifetime warranty, as in the case of a muffler, nor can a client return defective merchandise as she can in the case of a clothing store. Accountability in the human services comes from empirical practice.

Simple monitoring is a form of accountability in which we can begin to establish cause and effect. Social research is central to this thrust and research methods may be effectively applied in connection with direct practice and as Thomas (1975) notes, may provide critical information to be employed in working toward service objectives.

Evaluation of practice will not only satisfy the demands of third party funders and consumers, but it will provide the clinician with first hand information about her or his own practice (Gingerich, 1979). Empirical evidence can indicate which interventions work in different situations with different clients and allow practitioners to systematically accumulate the most effective practice modes.

Defining the Single Case Design

Single case research is the systematic observation of a specific behavior or set of behaviors over a period of time. The observation is expected to be standard in the measurement of behavior or activity. The observer may well be observing himself or herself (self monitoring) or someone else or some non-human target behavior activity (external monitoring). A schedule should be designed to include instruments to measure the observed target behavior. Copies of this schedule should be constructed in such a fashion that easy access be afforded the data collection process. The pattern created by these observations is analyzed for change through time and in relation to an introduced (intervening) or experimental variable. Single case designs include the major features of time series analysis which are common to the study of economic data. The experimental dimension is added when an intervening (experimental or treatment) variable "X" is introduced after the establishment of baseline behavior. The use of an intervening variable is optional and need not be planned or introduced at all. This distinguishes "monitor designs" from "single case designs." However, monitoring behavior tends to produce a change in behavior as a result of observing it. This is referred to

2

as "reactivity." This is sometimes a desired effect and is encouraged in certain kinds of enterprises such as weight loss programs and cigarette smoking reduction efforts. More often than not, the self-monitored behavior will be accompanied by a treatment or experimental variable. This will be followed by a period of continued observation and data collection of the target behavior or set of behaviors. The design is summarized in the following diagram.

Figure 1.

BASIC DESIGN

Experimental variable (counseling, treatment, etc.)

$$B_o \; B_o \; B_o \; B_o \; X \; A_o \; A_o \; A_o$$

B = observations before the introduction of X variable
A = observations after the introduction of X variable
X = experimental variable, etc.

Historical Review

A historical review is appropriate to understand and fully appreciate single subject designs. Modern psychology has always been associated with the study of the individual, however, experimental psychology and physiology during the middle of the nineteenth century is often cited as the beginning of experiments performed on individuals in basic research. The results of numerous N=1 studies were the origins of theories and constructs today. Hersen and Barlow (1976) present a concise history, much of which is summarized below.

"Broca's Area," the speech center of the brain, was discovered from a single case in which Paul Broca, in 1861, performed an autopsy on a patient hospitalized due to an inability to speak. His results were generalized and had a major impact on experimental psychology. Gustav Theodor Fechner (1801-1887) has been associated with the beginnings of experimental psychology with his publication of Elemente der Psychophysik, 1860. Fechner was a physiologist, physicist, psychophysicist, experimental estheticist, and philosopher during his

lifetime. He was one of the first to apply statistical
procedures to psychology problems, and was interested
in determining sensory thresholds of individuals. He
found that sensory thresholds varied within a subject
and the thresholds distributed themselves around a mean,
which characterized the true threshold. In other words,
a normal curve was applicable to variations within a
subject. Wilhelm Wundt, known as the first "psycholo-
gist," continued with the same single subject methodology as Fechner, in studying perception and sensation.
He established the first experimental psychological
laboratory. Perhaps because of these beginnings, a
strong tradition of studying individual organisms has
ensued in the fields of sensation, perception, and
physiological psychology.

Psychology students are usually introduced to the
subject of memory and retention by the results of Her-
man Ebbinghaus (1885), who was influenced by Fechner's
methods. He investigated the effect of different variables, such as the amount of material to be remembered,
on the efficiency of memory. He used a scientifically
derived self-monitoring design. Ebbinghaus' work established the pattern for much of the research on verbal learning during the past 80 years (Dukes, 1965).
Perhaps his best known discovery was the retention
curve, which illustrates the process of forgetting over
time. What is outstanding was his emphasis on repeated
measures of performance in one individual over time.

Pavlov's classical conditioning experiments (1928)
were single case experimental designs. He made a major
contribution to the principles of association and
learning, yet his methodology is often overlooked.
Cannon and Washburn's experiment with hunger and food
seeking behavior (1912) yielded new information in the
area of motivation. After swallowing a balloon, Washburn's stomach contractions were shown to coincide with
his introspective reports of hunger pangs (Dukes, 1965).

The landmark cases in the development of psychology
have been single case experimental designs. However,
during the late nineteenth century, another approach
arose due to the influence of Charles Darwin and Adolphe
Quetelet.

The Use of Statistics and Formation of the Group Comparison Approach

Adolphe Quetelet, in 1835, was the first to apply

the normal law of error to the distribution of human data, biological and social (Boring, 1950). His doctrine, l'homme moyen, described the "average" man as nature's ideal. The idea of mathematical treatment of the inheritance of genius was one that Quetelet suggested to Galton.

However, ten years earlier, in 1859, Charles Darwin published The Origin of Species, which is considered by many to be the greatest scientific advancement of the nineteenth century. It was Darwin's influence on Galton, his half cousin, that led to the interest of measuring individual mental inheritance. But, as we know, Darwin was interested in the variability within a species.

In 1901, Galton, Pearson, and Weldon founded the journal, Biometrika, for mathematical researchers in biology and psychology (Boring, 1950). Many of the newly devised statistical tests were published in that journal. Karl Pearson was often more enthusiastic about the statistics than the research problem.

In 1904, Galton began research in eugenics at the University of London with a concern to improve the human race. Later Karl Pearson was granted a research fellowship at The Francis Galton Laboratory of National Eugenics. Pearson's work on statistical methods, especially the present mathematical foundation of correlation, led to factor analysis, which was developed by Thurstone in the 1930's, and significant advances in construction of intelligence tests first introduced by Binet in 1905.

Concern for differences among individuals led to comparing groups by means of the newly developed descriptive statistics. From 1900 to 1930, much of the research in experimental psychology took advantage of these statistics to compare groups of subjects on various performance tests. Crude statistics that could attribute differences between groups to something other than chance began to appear, such as the critical ratio test.

R. A. Fisher, a name associated with the analysis of variance, succeeded Pearson at the Galton Laboratory in London. Fisher worked with the notions of induction and inference, or generalizing the findings to a larger problem. Fisher worked out the properties of statistical tests, which made it possible to estimate the rele-

vance of data from one small group with certain characteristics to the universe of individuals with those
characteristics. Because now it was possible to infer
from sample to population from the developments in
sampling theory, the single subject study lost popular-
ity. Psychological research insisted upon group comparisons and statistical estimation. Although B. F.
Skinner was working on operant conditioning, his work
did not make an impact on the present methodology,
since applied research was just beginning to develop.

Theories based on successful cases were constructed
and shared among therapists and soon the various schools
of psychotherapy were formed. The case-study method
(a forefather of today's single case experiments) was
the sole methodology of clinical investigation through
the first half of the twentieth century. However, this
method did not utilize the principles of applied research, such as definition of variables and manipulation of independent variables. Clinicians simply reported their successful findings, although some of the
more famous case studies were more scientific and systematic.

For example, Watson and Rayner's infamous study of
Albert's being conditioned to fear a white rat has been
cited as one of the most influential papers in the history of American psychology (Dukes, 1965). Breuer's
and Freud's treatment of Anna O. is analogous to a multiple baseline single subject design; although the variables were not clearly defined, the treatment was effective. However, due to the abundance of successful
case studies, with each school of thought boasting their
own success, applied researchers were reluctant to
accept case studies as valid indicators of effective
treatment since many of the case studies were uncon-
trolled and their results exaggerated. This had a
detrimental effect on the growth of experimental single
case designs.

What then followed in applied research was the
between-group comparisons and percentage of reported
success with certain treatments. However, since all
kinds of treatments showed some improvement, those ad-
vocating a certain treatment continued to publicize
their theories over others. The group comparison approach had many limitations and, as a result, many
studies were misleading, such as Eysenck's assertion
that psychotherapy is ineffective with neurotics. The
averaging of results (some better, some worse) cancelled

out any net effect since Eysenck only reviewed statistical findings. What was then realized was that such broad categories as "psychotherapy" and "neurotic" must be operationally defined into variables.

Two approaches, naturalistic and process studies, were advanced since many researchers were wondering if meaningful research could be done in regard to the evaluation of psychotherapy.

However, naturalistic studies lacked control and the power to isolate effects by its very nature of being a correlational study. The "flight into process" research so often cited appealed to clinicians because the therapeutic process was studied for individual patients and scientists were pleased that variables could be defined more precisely. Unfortunately, a polarization resulted between "process" and "outcome" studies. The former obtained measures during the treatment and the latter obtained pre and post measures via the group comparison method. This reluctance to relate process variables to outcome and the resulting inability of this approach to evaluate the effects of psychotherapy led to a decline of process research (Hersen and Barlow, 1976). Naturalistic studies and group comparisons did not provide an effective method for evaluating clinical practice.

Bergin and Strupp, in 1970, proposed in a paper, "New Directions in Psychotherapy Research," that the experimental single case approach be used for the purpose of isolating mechanisms of change in the therapeutic process. It was argued that the science of psychology should attend to the uniqueness of the individual. Shapiro's early work during the 1950's on the scientific investigation of individuals was largely ignored. He utilized carefully constructed measures of clinically relevant responses administered repeatedly over time in an individual.

The rediscovery of the experimental single case first occurred in basic research in physiology in 1957. Claude Bernard, a noted physiologist, persuaded his colleagues that the scientific study of the individual is only logical because group averages and variances are too misleading. The intensive scientific study of the individual in physiology then flourished. In applied research this approach was coupled with an emerging approach known as behavior modification therapy. However, single case methodology and behavior therapy

7

are not synonymous. The relevance of the experimental analysis of behavior to applied research is the development of sophisticated methodology enabling intensive study of individual subjects. With single case methods, one can begin to answer the question, "What specific treatment is effective with what type of client under what circumstances?"

The Purpose of Single Case Methodologies

The purpose of single case designs lies in their utility as a powerful tool for both practitioner and client to aid in the problem identification and problem solving process. Single case designs are not a substitute for good therapy, casework, or counseling, but instead function as a medium through which social work practice can be approached. In fact, the use of single case designs will no doubt highlight a successful practice or point to weaknesses that a practitioner may not be aware of.

Single case methodology is really a generic term which implies an approach to practice, and not a certain theory or treatment modality; thus, there are numerous types of single case designs a practitioner can implement. Moreover, this approach may enable a practitioner to increase her or his efficiency and productivity by the information and knowledge generated. With an empirical mode of operation one can become more aware of effects and causes, or determining influences on behavior or emotions.

Once again, as mentioned earlier in the historical review, this methodology is not new, but rather is being rediscovered and improved for the purpose of overall accountability, the improvement of practitioner functioning, and most importantly, the improvement of services to clients.

The practitioner may choose a single case monitoring design as a tool for problem identification and assessment, first of all, to increase client and practitioner awareness of an activity, behavior, instance, or event. In addition, monitoring may provide information as to the volume of time involved in a given activity or may help to identify more precisely the pattern of occurrence of an event. In many cases, a client may identify a presenting problem, and yet not be cognizant of the source, in which case monitoring

8

may be invaluable.

Some practitioners find that utilizing an N=1 empirical approach to their practice may actually aid in the treatment or intervention itself. For example, asking a client to monitor her feelings after an argument with her spouse may produce a heightened consciousness of those feelings. This is referred to as reactivity and this alone may be desirable for some clients. Basic to the purpose of N=1 is to find effective interventions, in order to change behaviors, processes, activities, or feelings, depending on the situation.

Single case designs facilitate staff development as practitioners become more aware and systematic in the treatment process. With this, we can validate the effectiveness of any type of treatment, document client change, further the social work knowledge base, and at the same time evaluate practice. However, as Scott Briar (in Jayaratne and Levy, 1979) notes:

> It is tempting to offer some drastic predictions about the wonderful things these clinical-research methods will make possible, but it is best not to promise too much too soon. It is sufficient, for the present, to say that even if only a small fraction of practitioners make use of the methods described in this book (Empirical Clinical Practice), social work and related fields will have taken a major step in the direction of demonstrating and increasing the effectiveness of their clinical activities.

Still, the strengths of single case research are in its flexibility, implementation, and the final product or the new knowledge generated.

One can utilize most treatment modalities or theoretical orientations, and one can use the method with individuals, couples, families, groups, or systems. The method is tailored to each case and thus is consistent with a social work philosophy which seeks to enhance the uniqueness of the individual. In other words, social work practice and single subject designs are not antithetical to one another. The criterion focus of practice fits well within a single case design. And likewise, one is not sacrificing research ideals by varying the kind of intervention at different times. In many senses, what the single case framework

9

calls for social workers should already practice: careful assessment, problem identification and intervention.
These phases are an integral part of social work practice and single subject designs.

Training to use single subject methods need not
be extensive and the method is usually simple to admin-
ister with most clients. The information yield is both
specific to the individual client and yet it is possible to group similar clients, problems, or interventions
and generalize findings. For example, one could accumulate single cases for nomothetic purposes.

Analysis of the data collected can be easily eye-
balled or even computerized. A variety of techniques
for analyzing data have been developed, which yield
information not only useful to practitioners and clients, but useful to social agencies for evaluative
purposes. These techniques require no more tools than
a pocket calculator and graph paper.

Single subject research, not being new, does not
mean it has been perfected. Although its potential
has hardly been realized, there are limitations inherent in self-observation. Problems with reliability and
instrumentation obviously should not be ignored. Addi-
tionally, how do we measure covert data? On the practical side, are not practitioners burdened with enough
"paperwork"? Bloom and Fisher (1982) present an excellent discussion on these issues and present them as
basic issues regarding single system designs. They are
certainly worthwhile considerations, yet we feel the
benefits outweigh the costs.

CHAPTER 2

RESEARCH DESIGNS FOR TESTING INTERVENTION

Introduction

In this chapter we want to examine the issue of
research design as it pertains to the testing of hypotheses using the single case approach. In order to do
this we will: (1) compare the single case approach
with the group approach or ideographic with the nomothetic, (2) examine the relation of single case designs
with the traditional research designs, (3) explain the
use and meaning of monitoring and the several designs
that spring from the monitoring process, (4) compare a
variety of commonly used single case designs, (5) illustrate multiple baseline designs, (6) review the
critical threats to the validity of single case studies,
(7) discuss the problems of generalizability for single
case studies, and last, (8) examine the "appropriate-
ness" of certain designs over others.

It should be made very clear at this point that
the research design is most important to understand
because it establishes the logical basis for comparing
and evaluating the information being studied. Of all
the activities of research the most critical activity
that makes science science and giving it validity is
"observation." Observation is central to scientific
integrity. Research design is the arrangement of
these observations and how these observations occur.
To put it another way, research design is the juxtaposi-
tion of observations and dominated by the temporal
factor. . .the passage of time.

Before we go further with the issue of design of
research studies, we must understand first the similar-
ities and differences between single case research and
group comparison research. Almost all of us have been
schooled in the use and sometimes misuse of statistical
techniques. Statistical analysis is, of course, applied
to the groups of cases or observations anywhere from a
half dozen to thousands of cases. But when we employ
a single case design we are studying only one (n=1)
case (but many observations). Most of us have done
counseling and/or casework and know the method for
studying and understanding one client. This approach
is qualitative and is valued very highly among those of
the helping professions. The quantitative approach is

11

not concerned with the integrity of the individual but more concerned with group characteristics such as average age, voting behavior of low income people, health conditions of new-born infants, etc. However, the single case approach gives one the ability to examine the individual as a unique being and as a member of a group or community. Let us examine a few of the most important issues involved in the study of individuals and groups of individuals.

Comparison of Single Case Analysis with Group Comparison Analysis

We are aiming to achieve in our work prediction and generalization. Generalization follows from successful prediction (Howe, 1974). However, we must answer the question, "Are we trying to generalize to individuals or to groups?"

If the premises are statistical in nature, only statements about classes of events may be either explained or predicted. If the premises are deterministic, we may predict an individual event. The purpose at hand should guide whether we are interested in applying the findings to individuals or groups.

Statistical and deterministic premises are not directly comparable. Statistical premises are actuarial where the prediction attempts to say, "most persons of this type will respond in X manner to Y treatment." This type of prediction has applied value for the program administrator or planner. The clinician, however, wants to be able to predict relationships between specific environmental interventions and behaviors of single individuals (Browning and Stover, 1971).

Nomothetic propositions are made for groups or a general class of events (all teenagers, for example) with statistical predictions, while idiographic propositions are made for individual events with deterministic predictions.

Individual-Control/Applied-Analysis Strategy is the type of analysis associated with single case designs. Data is collected only from one individual over extended periods of time; in group comparison approaches data are collected over a short period of time and grouped into control and experimental groups. In single case (subject) designs, the individual serves

12

as his own control and experimental analysis (visual inspection of data points) is substituted for statistical analysis. By obtaining a <u>steady state</u>, a situation in which the characteristics of the phenomenon under observation do not change over a period of time, such as the frequency of intoxication, arguments or headaches, experimental control is achieved and can easily be translated into practice. For example, if uncontrollable anger is a problem for the client, the practitioner can locate the specific conditions or occasions when his anger occurs (Howe, 1974). This establishment of the steady state then is amenable for change and the worker is attuned as to where to begin.

Control-Group/Statistical-Analysis Strategy is the type of analysis with group designs where control groups, statistical analysis, and significance tests are used (Howe, 1974). This strategy may still be of interest to the social worker who is interested in the analysis of groups and group behavior. The U.S. census data is a good example of grouped data of great value to planners. Also, agency statistics are vital to an agency's justification of budget when applying for funding. The ideographic or single case approach provides a very different kind of data, that being essentially change experienced by a single entity.

Overview of Research Designs

Figure 2 shows the reader an overall view of the major research designs. These designs--survey, experimental, and quasi-experimental--represent the most common designs used by most researchers today. It should be noticed that survey designs have been divided into two subtypes: cross-sectional and longitudinal. Survey research refers to observations which have been made at one time only without any acknowledgement of a cause-effect connection. The cross-sectional design focuses on one time only studies such as exploratory, where hypotheses are to be developed from one's exploration. The descriptive studies, such as the formal community type study, attempts to answer questions about how many, how much, where, why, and when (the U.S. census is a good example of a descriptive survey). Explanatory studies have all the characteristics of descriptive studies, but go further by attempting to establish causal or relational connections between survey variables. Longitudinal surveys refer to studies that are repeated two or more times (using the same

Figure 2.

RESEARCH DESIGNS

Survey		Experimental	Quasi-Experimental
Cross Sectional	Longitudinal	Group Comparison	Single-Case Designs
Exploratory	Trend	Before & After	Baseline, Treatment, Withdrawal
Descriptive	Cohort	Before & After (No control)	A B A
Explanatory	Panel	Before & After 1 & After 2	A B A B
		Before & After 1 & After 2 (w/control)	A B C A
		After Only	A B A B A
		After Only w/control	
		Solomon Four Group	

14

instruments). The trend longitudinal design takes samples regarding issues two or more times with different groups of individuals very much in the manner of the national polls. The cohort studies do the same, except they sample within a given sub-population; that is, subsequent smaller sub-samples are taken on successive occasions into the future. The panel designs do the same, only the researcher continues to return to the same subjects each successive sampling time.

The experimental designs refer to the traditional meaning of that concept; that is, observations at one time followed by an intervention and a second observation. The classical experimental design adds a control group where the intervention is not introduced. Comparisons are then made of the two groups at time two, as can be seen in Figure 3.

Figure 3.

CLASSICAL EXPERIMENTAL DESIGN

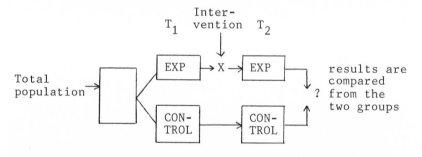

The experimental designs in Figure 2 may vary in the degree of control but the time factor and the presence of an intervention are critical features to the definition of such designs.

Many researchers have defined more carefully as to what makes a design experimental and what doesn't. The important difference to most writers is the presence or absence of a control group. Where there is no control group researchers have tended to label such designs as quasi-experimental. It is at this point that single case designs become associated with experimental research. Because of the presence of a deliberately introduced intervention, single case designs may be

15

considered experimental.

Monitoring Designs

As discussed in the first chapter, the study of single units has been going on for as long as the analysis of group data. The observation of single units through time is a common characteristic of many different kinds of research efforts. The mere fact that researchers have observed on a regular and systematic basis phenomena provides the essential character of all experimental work. This process is called monitoring and it is common to all kinds of everyday activity for the primary purpose of determining the direction of behavior and the changing quality of phenomena. The ever illusive quality of change can only be detected by making occasional observations to measure a phenomenon for the same attributes as observed at a previous time. In the manufacture of products monitoring is referred to as quality control. The night watchman, like the military sentry, monitors for unauthorized activity in a given area. Monitoring specific social problems produces social indicators that are absolutely necessary for planning for social needs.

Below in Figure 4 a wide range of monitoring designs are indicated. This figure emphasizes the notion that many different kinds of studies of single units require monitoring. There are at least five branches or sub-variations of the more general design or process

Figure 4.

MONITOR DESIGNS

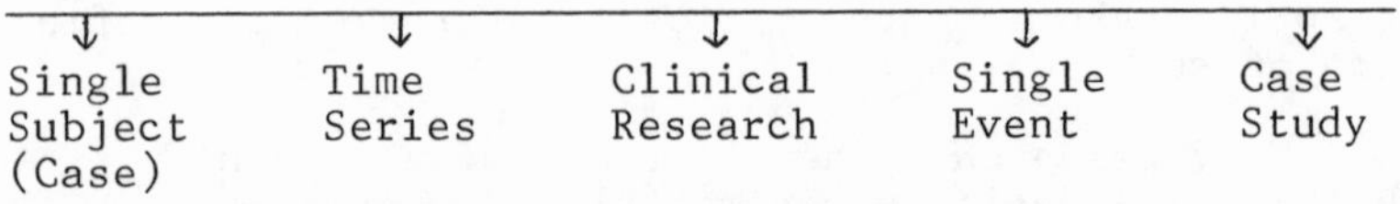

↓	↓	↓	↓	↓
Single Subject (Case)	Time Series	Clinical Research	Single Event	Case Study

called monitoring. As indicated, monitoring is a broader, more inclusive concept than single subject, time series, single case, case study, and clinical research. Time series is common to economic activity through time. Single subject is a label commonly used by clinical psychologists and used interchangeably with

16

"single case." Both refer to the study of individuals, although it could be in reference to the study of auto performance, or social groups, or movie house attendance. "Case studies" refer to the social worker's analysis of a client's problem by means of examining the interrelationship of various life factors to understand the client's presenting behavior. Finally, clinical research refers to the study of clients as a process without focusing on a time one, intervention, and time two outcome. Clinical research is primarily concerned with process and relationship of therapist and client through time. But let us now give our attention to the most popular and common sub-variations, single case designs.

Single Case Designs

As described in the first chapter, the "method" can be seen as a T_1 (time one), X (intervention) and T_2 (time two) or outcome. This design is the most common of all designs used by researchers and practitioners. It is normally referred to as an "A-B-A" design: "A" meaning baseline, "B" as intervention or treatment, and "A" referred to as baseline (again) or withdrawal. The second most common, especially in field practice, is the "A-B," where only a baseline and intervention is employed. The following set of illustrations show each of five designs that are used by most researchers. Small boxes (□) are to denote baseline and X is to denote intervention/treatment. The dots represent the daily observation of some activity (dependent variable). It should be remembered that there are more combinations that can be invented dependent upon the needs of the study situation. For example, one can introduce and withdraw numerous treatment modalities over a long period of time. But it is sufficient to examine these five to converge the variety of possibilities.

Figure 5.

"B" DESIGN

This is the most elementary of all designs.

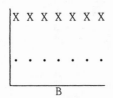

No baseline, treatment only. Monitor through time
with objective measures taken repeatedly. Case study
method, observe for a series of variables. There is
little or no control over variables. One may consider
this design as no design at all, yet it is quite common among treatment practitioners.

Figure 6.

"A-B" DESIGN

This is a rather common design for practitioners.
(2 phases).

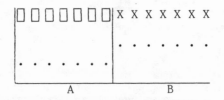

Baseline and treatment; treatment not withdrawn,
continued for clinical reasons. This is the simplest
form of the experimental designs. "A" phase, natural
development of the target behavior under study. "B"
phase, treatment is introduced and changes in the dependent variable are noted. Reservations: (1) changes
might have occurred anyway, (2) they may be correlated
with an event.

Figure 7.

"A-B-A" DESIGN

This design is becoming more common among practitioners. (3 phases.)

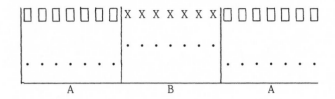

Baseline, treatment, withdrawal. If after baseline "A" measurements of dependent (target variable) are taken and treatment or intervention is applied "B" leads to improvement and subsequently back to deterioration after it is withdrawn "A," we can feel confident that the intervention had something to do with the change. Limitation: if giving treatment it would be unethical to stop treatment for client.

Figure 8.

"A-B-A-B" DESIGN

This design is highly recommended by researchers. (4 phases.)

```
|□ □ □ □ □ □ □|X X X X X X X|□ □ □ □ □ □ □|X X X X X X X
|            |  . . . . . .|            |  . . . . . . .
|            |            |            |
|. . . . . . |            | . . . . . . |
|_____|_____|_____|_____
      A            B            A              B
```

Baseline-treatment-withdrawal and treatment. This eliminates the problem of ethical considerations in ABA. It also further verifies the effectiveness of treatment.

Figure 9.

"A-B-BC-B" DESIGN

This design makes use of variations in the intervention variable. (4 phases.)

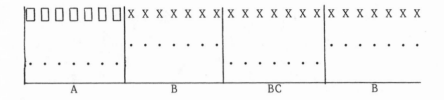

Baseline, treatment #1 treatment #1 & treatment #2, treatment #1. This BC introduction means simultaneous introduction of treatment believed to be more effective than if introduced sequentially.

Multiple Baseline Designs

Up to this point we have been concerned with the study of one client with one problem and one intervention. As we have seen, most involve a baseline, intervention and withdrawal. Multiple baseline designs give the researcher the opportunity to examine the impact of an intervention on more than one client, more than one situation, and more than one problem. That is, multiple baseline designs make use of a sequentially applied intervention to two or more problems, situations or individuals. Comparisons and contrasts can be made using this design that cannot be made using single dimension designs such as AB, ABA or ABAB. Also, frequently it is not desirable to remove the intervention because it is having a positive effect for a client. In such cases a multiple baseline is valuable because no reversal (withdrawal) is necessary to determine the impact of the intervention.

There are three common multiple designs that we will discuss here. Each design deals with multiple problems or multiple individuals or multiple situations. It should be remembered that in each example the same intervention is used.

In Figure 10 a multiple baseline has been set up

Figure 10.

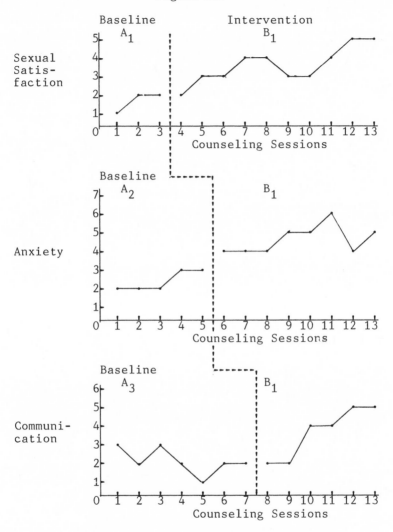

for testing the impact of counseling on three different problems of one client. This is called a multiple
baseline across <u>problems</u>. The counselor works with the
client regarding sexual satisfaction after baseline of
three sessions has been established. After some success in this problem area the counselor focuses the
counseling on anxiety of the client and later still the
counselor focuses on the problem of communication of
the client. As can be seen, baseline data are gathered
on all three problems from the beginning of the case.
As can be seen, counseling was effective in all three
areas.

    In the event that the counselor is working with
two clients with a similar problem such as drug abuse
a multiple baseline can be applied to test the impact
of counseling in regard to "communication with family"
(see Figure 11).

Figure 11.

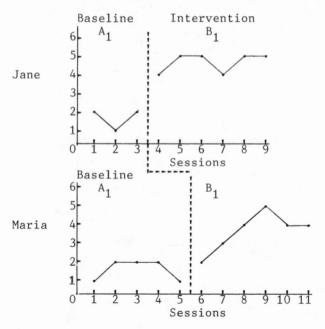

The scale is given each counseling session to both clients. The counseling regarding "communication with family" is focused first on Jane after three sessions of baseline was established. Later counseling in the same area is focused on Marie. As can be seen, counseling was effective because it shows a clear difference between the third session for Jane and the fifth session for Maria; that is, Maria remained low during the time Jane improved.

In the case of using multiple baseline designs in different situations we can set up the experiment by selecting a client who is a youth with behavior difficulty and is coming to the agency for counseling. Figure 12 shows the counselor's graphs where the coun-

Figure 12.

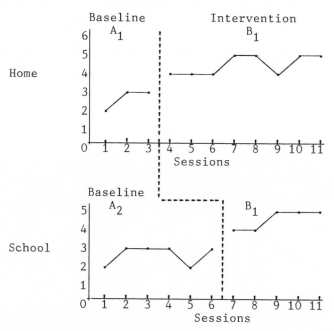

seling is focused on first behavior at home and later on, behavior at school after an initial period of baseline data regarding negative behaviors without specific counseling. The graphs show that the counseling intervention was effective regardless of the situation.

Finally, it can be seen that multiple baselines can be very useful in testing the external validity of an intervention (generalizability) which is the weakest issue in the use of single case designs discussed earlier.

One last approach should be mentioned before leaving design types and that is the testing of multiple baselines for more than one problem without withholding the intervention from several problems while focused on one at a time. That is, the clinician-researcher may simply want to see what impact a general intervention may have on a series of problems. This "carry over" effect may tell the worker something of the relation between and among problem areas that are similarly effected by a common intervention.

The Validity of Experiments

There are numerous problems with single case designs but the most worrisome has to do with validity. A perfect experiment would be composed of an experimental group and a control group. Both groups would be created as a result of randomly assigning cases to each. The critical issue would be to establish internal validity or causality. Establishing causality requires that all factors be ruled out as rival explanations of the observed association between the intervention and target (problem) behavior. It is asking a lot to achieve such purity but it can be done if the threats to validity are observed. Campbell and Stanley, in their now classic book on experimental designs (Campbell and Stanley, 1963), enumerate eight threats to validity. They are worth reporting here as a guide to practitioners who strive for perfection but fall short in the uncontrollable environment of social service agencies.

The threats to the internal validity of experiments are as follows:

1. History--the events that happen to occur from the first observation or test to the second that are not related to the introduced intervention. For example, a woman client who is in counseling terminates her case after her husband has returned to the family. Was it the returning husband or the counseling that

24

effected the termination?

2. Maturation--the processes within the client which occur as a natural function of the passing of time such as growing older. For example, the study of pre-school children over time where the intervention is learning skills. Did the children achieve skills as a result of the pre-school program or as a result of merely growing older?

3. Experimental mortality--the loss of subjects during the life of the experiment. The results could be altered because of this loss and not the counseling.

4. Instrumentation--changes in the measurements from time one to time two or changes in scoring procedures. The researcher cannot determine if the results are due to the intended intervention or the differences in the measurements and scoring methods.

5. Testing--the effects of taking a test upon the scores of a time two testing. That is, when the same scale of measure is used for both T_1 and T_2 the subject will have gained some experience with the test the first time. The question is: are the results due to previous experience with the test or the intervention?

6. Differential selection--in experiments with an experimental and control group subjects in one group may be different from those in the second group. If this is true then the results of the experiment may be due to this difference and not the intervention.

7. Statistical regression--this threat results from selecting a subject or subjects from an extreme situation. For example, individuals coming to counseling who are involved in a divorce will over time very likely return to a normal emotional state. In such cases the end results may be due to normality returning to the client rather than the intervention of counseling.

8. Selection/Maturation interaction--one of the comparison groups may be more mature than the other. For example, if the experimental group is made up of older clients, compared to the control group which might be made up of younger clients. The maturation difference may well be effecting the outcome of the experiment and not the interaction.

The single case experiment has many serious problems, but the issue of control group being important is dealt with in that the case or subject serves as his own control by means of the design or ABA, baseline, intervention and withdrawal. That is, data being taken on the subject during intervention is then observed during withdrawal. On many occasions clinicians may be working with two or more clients with the same problem, very much like the multiple baseline design across individuals and provides control over some variables.

Variability and Generalizability

As clinicians and/or researchers, we must be concerned with the variability and generality of the data. We accept the fact that our behavior is a function of many social factors. We hope to be able to say that the treatment introduced has caused a change in behavior. But what about all those variables that may impact on the case besides the intervention variable?

In group designs variability is removed by control of a variable in the experimental design. That is, a control group is present for comparison purposes at time one and at time two. In single case research, the practitioner could accommodate himself to the variability with immediate alteration in experimental design to test out hypothesized sources of these changes (Hersen and Barlow, 1976). The practitioner can use repeated measures of the problem behavior and can also change the experimental design to locate sources of variability. However, a judgement must be made as to how much behavioral variability to ignore when looking for functional relations among overall trends in behavior and the treatment in question (Hersen and Barlow, 1976). Because we want to determine the effects of a given treatment, we may not wish to change the design midway through (the more pragmatic strategy)(Hersen and Barlow, 1976).

In experimental designs such as A-B-A-B, where one is looking for cause and effect relationships, investigators will occasionally resort to averaging two data points within a phase, which is sometimes called blocking (Hersen and Barlow, 1976). This does not remove the variability; it simply makes trends more apparent. However, all points should be analyzed so that other practitioners can draw their own conclusions.

Large intra-subject variability is
a common feature during repeated measurements of target behavior in a single case,
particularly in the beginning of an experiment when the subject may be accommodating
to intrusive measures. How much variability is the researcher willing to tolerate
before introducing a therapeutic procedure
is largely a question of judgement on the
part of the investigator (Hersen and Barlow,
1976).

The results can be more generalizable if more
sources of variability are located. Experience has
taught us that precision or control leads to more extensive generalization of data (Sidman, 1960). Generalization usually pertains to:

1. generality of findings across subjects or
   clients
2. generality across practitioners
3. generality across settings

To a great extent these forms of generality are
achieved by multiple baseline designs. Generalizations
to other individuals are based on logical considerations. Once a significant difference appears within
the single case, one can specify the particular client
background variables and other relevant characteristics
in which the significant result was actually obtained
(Chassan, 1961).

Replication of studies is probably the only agreed
upon method to demonstrate generality. Edgar and Billingsley (1974) describe three types of replication.
They are:

1. literal replication (same practitioner,
   same intervention)
2. operational replication (other practitioners,
   same intervention)
3. constructive replication (vary procedure
   but verify identical relationships)

Choosing an Appropriate Design

Edwin Thomas (1975) has made a distinction between
"fixed intervention strategy" and "criterion-oriented"
methods of clinical evaluation. This distinction may

27

aid the practitioner in choosing a design. By a fixed intervention we mean an intervention which has been employed previously and is being used now to further test the intervention strategy (independent variable). That is, an intervention that does not emerge during the baseline phase of the study.

The criterion-oriented strategy is explicitly concerned with outcome and provides feedback to clients and practitioners. This strategy also yields information on the independent variable, but is less rigorous than the fixed intervention (Jayaratne, Levy, 1979). The advantage of the criterion-oriented strategy is that it may be used in a much more pragmatic manner. The worker and client may decide late in the therapy that a new intervention should be tried without returning to baseline after the application of an ineffective intervention. The more classical researcher would not be so tempted. He/she would remain with the first intervention and move directly to a withdrawal (second baseline) phase to determine if withdrawal is comparable to baseline 1. The comparison of Baseline 1 to Intervention 1 to Withdrawal 1 provides the final proof of intervention effectiveness. Again, the therapist may feel much more comfortable with the design that yields to the demands of the therapist-client relationship.

CHAPTER 3

PROBLEM DEFINITION AND
INDEPENDENT-DEPENDENT VARIABLES

Overview

Single case studies can be carried out under a variety of circumstances. If, for example, one is trying to reduce the number of cigarettes one smokes it does not require a laboratory or special equipment to carry on the project. More important is the character of this problem in terms of its complexity; that is, every problem that human service workers encounter is really a complex of many factors that push and pull upon the individual whether he or she likes it or not. The social worker in the one-to-one treatment setting takes a social history or a means of getting a fix on the complex of problems in order to find what the levels of pain, fear, anxiety, strength may be for the client. Out of this effort comes a treatment plan to begin removing blocks to making choices for more satisfactory functioning. This means understanding and perhaps monitoring a series of problems, monitoring them in order to determine their interrelationship and interplay. From this approach we can best determine how to attack specific problems and reduce their pressure on the client.

The first step can be thought of as assessment, a procedure by which the practitioner identifies and empirically characterizes the presenting problems, with their related situational and social psychology factors, and the goals of intervention. The goals of intervention follow almost automatically as one learns of the problem or problems to be attacked. The aim of assessment is to help the client and practitioner determine the target problems for intervention and determine intervention goals (Jayaratne and Levy, 1979).

The target problem and related goal must be identified and Jayaratne and Levy suggest the criteria offered by Sundel (in Jayaratne and Levy, 1979) for selecting a priority problem for intervention. These suggestions are especially helpful at this early stage in the experimental process. Sundel suggests:

1. Select the problem that is the immediate concern of the client or significant others.

2. Select the problem that has the most aversive consequences to the individual, significant others, or society. That is, minimize the pain that may be inflicted on self or others by the external situation.

3. Select the problem that can be corrected most quickly. Such a selection would give the client a successful experience in therapy, resulting in increased motivation and trust in the practitioner.

4. Select a problem that must be dealt with before any other problem can be resolved.

Once the target problem has been selected other secondary problems or observations may also be included in the monitoring process. The data collection schedule should be designed to make for easy collection of the necessary information. This phase of single case research will be examined at length later. The target problem and the secondary problems that presumably cluster around it should be operationally defined in order to make them as concrete in meaning as possible. This meaning, of course, should be related to the every day experience of these problems so that they may be observed and recorded with accuracy and reliability. The issue of reliability will be also examined in the following chapter.

Before we examine some common target problems we must first remind the reader that there is a focus to each single case study. This focus is called a <u>unit of analysis</u>.

Unit of Analysis

The unit of analysis is the recipient of our attention who will presumably benefit from the change in the target problems as a result of the introduction of the intervention. This unit of analysis is sometimes referred to as unit of study and could be an individual who might monitor himself. If one individual monitors another individual then the observed individual would be the unit of analysis. These individuals come in a wide variety, such as patients, clients, teenagers, foster parents, adoptive parents, students, husbands, wives, etc. It is equally possible to study a group such as a family, social group, friendship group; each would be considered a unit of analysis. Social groups lead by a professional practitioner can have her/his group evaluate itself after each meeting and then use the collected data to gain further insight into the dynamics of the group before introducing an intervention. A time study within an agency to increase lagging productivity (target problem) would make the agency the unit of analysis. Monitoring the use of play areas would make the play area (situation) the unit of analysis.

Target Problems (the Dependent Variable)

The list of target problems below are taken from those studies encountered by the authors' experience in working with undergraduates, graduates, workshop participants and community residents. More problems could be added but this list will suffice to inspire the reader with the notion that single case studies are endless in types and kinds of problems possible to study and overcome. The reader may want to add his/her own ideas to the list--do so--the list is meant to only suggest possibilities. But it is important to comment on some of those listed because of special problems that tend to arise as a result of their study. These comments are, of course, based on experience with over two hundred subjects over the last four years. A few comments should give the reader some idea of the common problems encountered.

The goal of weight reduction is a good example of the problem of poor achievement results but very positive behavior. This is a very popular target problem but few persons ever achieve significant change because weight loss is much too slow for a 30 to 40 day study. There has to be an unrealistic amount of weight loss to show a significant change. That is, there may be and usually is a substantial weight loss using single case methods but it doesn't show up. If the researcher uses calorie count instead of pounds significance will show positive results. The method is therefore very valuable in controlling weight with "maintenance" as a goal.

Cigarette smoking is almost always easy to reduce using the single case approach partly because cigarettes are well defined units that can be accurately observed on a daily basis.

Anxiety is difficult to measure but is a problem most people seem to bring under control using the method.

31

TARGET PROBLEMS

(The Dependent Variable)

Behaviors to be Monitored

1. Weight (reduce or increase)
2. Cigarette smoking (decrease)
3. Use of obscene language (reduce instant)
4. Telephone calls (increase positive use)
5. Supervisory interaction (increase confidence)
6. Sexual behavior (increased satisfaction)
7. Marital conflict (reduced)
8. Anger (instances of feeling)
9. Drinking alcohol (reduced consumption)
10. Buying and/or shopping (control spending)
11. Child-parent interaction (increase positive contact)
12. Ulcer attack (reduce)
13. Gallstone attack (reduce)
14. Exercising (increase)
15. Traffic (reduce frustration)
16. Sleeping (reduce hours of sleep)
17. Interpersonal contact (expressiveness-irritableness)
18. Study habits (increase school work completed)
19. Shyness (becoming more aggressive)
20. Childhood discipline (reduce instances)
21. Coffee consumption (reduce consumption)
22. Eye contact (increase)
23. Fear (of being alone, height, open space: reduce)
24. Number of daily accomplishments (increase)
25. Drinking (soft drinks: reduce)
26. Assertiveness
27. Interaction with co-workers (increase positive

contact)
28. Use of time (increase positive use)
29. Drugs (reduce dependence)
30. Procrastination (reduce)
31. Lateness (reduce or eliminate)
32. Treatment-therapy (maintain)
33. Daily management of duties (maintain)
34. Moodiness (decrease)
35. Use of medication (reduce dependence)
36. Study behavior (positive use of time)
37. Pain (relieve)
38. Diet (maintain)
39. Argumentation (reduce instances)
40. Television watching (reduce number of hours)
41. Aggression (reduce)
42. Class attendance (increase)
43. Reading speed (increase pages read)
44. Acts of aggression (reduce)
45. Number of times you say "yes" when you really mean "no"
46. Anxiety (reduce amount)
47. Embarrassment (reduce instances)
48. Morale (improve feeling)
49. Calories (maintain desired level)
50. Dependency on others (reduce occasions)

Ulcer and gallstone attacks do not occur very often, even for those who are chronically afflicted; that is, the time sweep must be very wide and therefore allowing a great deal of time between occasions for other (noise) events (history) to act as intervention instead of the intervention intended by the researcher-practitioner. It will be noted that practically all of those target problems listed are to be increased as an activity or reduced in its presence in the subject's life. It should also be noted that sometimes a target problem of one person (or the same person) may be used as an intervention for another person.

It is surprising how well and how confident people are in the faithful recording of data. Once the measure (of the target problem) has been established and defined there is rarely a problem with accurate measurement and recording. Let us leave this discussion in order to examine the issues involved in introducing the intervention.

The Intervention (the Independent Variable)

The introduction of the independent variable into the experimental management is a critical and exciting moment for the researcher. It is the time when one determines whether or not a cause-effect type of relationship exists between the independent variable and the dependent variable. In more traditional terms the independent variable is referred to as the "experimental" variable, or the "cause" variable or "treatment" variable or the "intervention" variable. From this point on we will use the term "intervention" as this seems to better suit many researchers and practitioners.

An intervention into an experiment is presumed to have some kind of impact on the target problem under question. That is, the goal of an intervention is of most interest to the practitioner-researcher for outcome or a criterion-oriented strategy is critical to helping clients achieve what they presumably come to the agency to find. . .(their goal) relief from some burdensome stress. It will be noted that the intervention is usually designed to do one of three things to the target problem: (1) reduce its effect on the subject, (2) increase its effect on the subject, (3) maintain the present level of its effect on the subject. Return to the list of target problems and one can see

34

that the great majority are concerned with reducing or increasing effect on the subject.

An intervention when applied to a target is "present" or when removed is "absent." This suggests that the experimenter should use care and discipline when applying the intervention: beginning at a precise time and concluding at a precise time. If the practitioner feels a needed intervention should be applied, so be it, but it should be introduced with discipline if its impact is to be clearly determined.

It should be mentioned at this point that in planning a single case study one should look to the literature in order to find adequate theory to connect the target problem and the planned intervention. All practitioners follow a practice theory or combination of theories that guide the treatment of her or his clients. Within this practice theory one must find justification for applying one intervention over another. This, of course, increases the chances of the intervention being successful in impacting on the target problem.

Beyond the simple AB or ABA designs interventions may be applied in a number of different and unique ways. <u>Multiple or successive intervention strategies</u> may be used to the advantage of the pragmatic practitioner. For example, an ABAB design means the same intervention is applied and removed and applied a second time in order to determine the precise effect of the intervention. Another design, such as AB_1AB_2 suggests that a second and different intervention has been introduced by the researcher-practitioner. This alternating of intervention and baseline can continue until success is experienced by the client. One other alternative is possible and useful; that is, an ABAC design where C represents maintenance. This is especially valuable where the client is successfully relieved of a stressful target problem and needs a regimen to continue present success.

It is not uncommon to find that several minor or secondary target problems are associated and even correlated with the primary target problem. The practitioner may see this correlation developing during the baseline or even after the first intervention has been applied. If so, one can take a secondary target problem and use it as an intervention with possible success. For example, coffee consumption may be moni-

tored as a secondary problem with sleep as the primary
target problem. When coffee consumption is removed
from the diet sleep comes sooner and more satisfactorily
to the client (patient).

The reinforcement of an intervention is also a
common occurrence in single case studies. More often
than not reinforcement means increasing or adding more
of the same to the client's situation. . .more exercise,
more sleep, more relaxation, more medication. Sometimes introducing the intervention more often during
the time sweep is helpful in producing the desired impact. In the case of multiple baseline across two or
more problems, the intervention is focused on first one
problem and then another and another as with counseling
fear of height, stress and communication with family
members. Counseling is the intervention but focused on
three different problems.

As was done with target problems, a series of
common interventions are listed below. These interventions are taken from the same studies that make up the
list of target problems discussed earlier in this chapter.

Unit of Observation or Time Sweep

Before leaving the subject of independent and
dependent variables, it is necessary to briefly discuss
the issue of time of observation or unit of observation. It is also commonly referred to as time sweep.
This refers to the time during which we are observing
for the target problem to manifest itself. This period
of time is not rigidly defined and prescribed, but is
dictated by the client's problem situation (Howe, 1974).
For example, the more frequent the target problem is
manifested the smaller the time unit necessary to observe the behavior of that problem. The more gross the
behavior of a problem the larger or longer the time
unit needs to be in order to observe its true character.
For example, an eye tic occurs many times during an
hour so the time sweep is an hour long and therefore
becomes the unit of observation. If the problem is
anger outbursts, which occur only a few times a day,
then the unit of observation should be one day. Here
are some suggestions:

One day? An hour? Twice a week? Every Friday?
Special days. . .i.e., pay day, visitation day, staff

36

INTERVENTIONS

(The Independent or Experimental Variable)

Condition to be Introduced

1. Relaxation exercises
2. Breathing exercises
3. Special diet program such as Weight Watchers
4. Calling friends
5. Self medication
6. Use of music
7. Friendly confessions
8. Therapy (group)
9. Therapy (individual)
10. Interval periods of rest
11. Grounding by parent
12. Meditation
13. Silence
14. Increase the amount of sleep
15. Ritual
16. Monitor behavior
17. Daily agenda (pre-monitoring)
18. Measure accomplishments by comparing your list with actual completed tasks
19. Play back taped material
20. Use recreation

meeting? During a moment? An event. . .i.e., family
gathering, meal time, sex. . .activity. . .bowling,
card games, group sessions?

Designing Hypotheses

We have been discussing the target problem and the
intervention in a single case study with care given to
the relationship between the two. Hopefully, a strong
theoretical connection exists to insure the success of
the experiment. However, one should understand that
this kind of research is only a variation on other more
traditional forms of research. Here, let's examine the
connection between the target or dependent variable and
the intervention or independent variable. Indeed, we
are speaking of variables as we do in survey and classic experimental work. In order to do this and make
clear the connection, we need to frame the study problem in traditional research terms which is, of course,
the hypothesis. Any research has as its core the hypothesis, which is to say, what do we expect to find?
What will be the outcome of this study? Let us start
by hypothesizing the outcome for an AB design. If we
hope to treat the alcoholic through counseling of some
kind then we might hypothesize that counseling will
reduce the amount of alcohol consumed. There are
other considerations in counseling such as employment,
family relations, use of money, but for now we wish to
begin to control the drinking behavior. The hypothesis
may be schematically designed as below in Figure 13.

Let us now test this hypothesis concerning alcohol
consumption by hypothetically carrying out a single
case study. In Figure 14 data have been reported by
the client before direct counseling and then after
counseling about drinking. The counseling seems to
have had some positive impact on the client. But let
us restructure Figure 14 into a traditional hypothesis
matrix as seen in Figure 15.

If this were data from a group, and if we were to
use the chi square technique for testing significant
differences, then our hypothesis would be tested as
significant, therefore providing evidence that counseling was effective in reducing alcohol consumption for
the client.

Let us examine this problem under the conditions
of no significant differences between counseling and no

38

Figure 13.

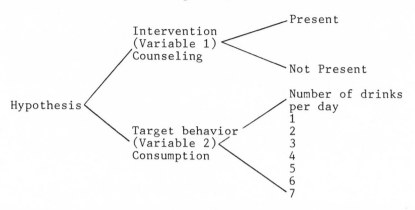

Figure 14.

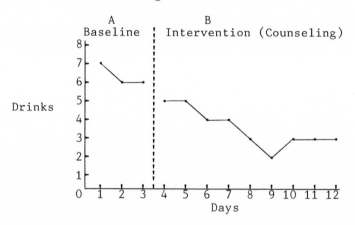

Figure 25.

HYPOTHESIS

		A No Counseling	B Counseling
Consumption	*High	X	
	Low		X

*We can define high and low by use of the median
number of drinks or an arbitrary number.

		A No Counseling	B Counseling
Consumption	High 5+	3	2
	Low 4-	0	7

counseling using the same hypothesis. In Figure 16
data have been gathered for a client before counseling
and after counseling had begun.

Figure 16.

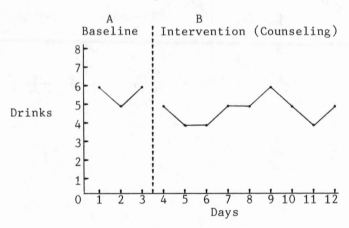

When the data have been tabulated by phase we see
no significant differences in the pattern.

40

Figure 17.

		A No Counseling	B Counseling
Consumption	High 5+	3	6
	Low 4-	0	3

It should be remembered that the pattern could be reversed with consumption being higher during counseling than before counseling, which would be a reverse of Figure 15.

One could continue to test hypotheses for ABA or ABAB designs using first AB and then BA and A_1A_2. The last test, A_1A_2, would be hypothesized as no significant difference since both phases are baseline and/or no counseling given.

CHAPTER 4

MEASUREMENT AND INSTRUMENTATION

Before we examine the issues of measurement it is important to clarify some of the terms we will be discussing in this chapter. For example, the term data collection schedule is almost always a set or series of instruments presented or given to respondents who respond to the questions and items therein. Collection schedule and instrument are not the same thing. An instrument is a tool or device used to measure a variable or phenomenon. The terms instrument and measurement are sometimes confused; that is, an instrument as a tool gives substance to a reality we think exists. A measurement is the consequence of a standardization of what we think is reality. The instrument gives the phenomenon a reality inasmuch as the instrument as substance and concreteness. For example, a 20 item scale which measures "coping" ability is made up of statements which, when responded to, reflect how a client feels in this area. The 20 items make up the instrument for measuring an illusive quality called "coping."

The Meaning of Measurement

If the products of instruments are measures of phenomena in and of reality what is measurement? Measurement is the objectification of reality and thereby giving it substance that can be viewed similar by many different observers. In the process of measurement the phenomena or reality is particularized in greater and greater specificity, i.e., 20 items of the "coping" scale. It also means that a detailed point of reference has been established from which many different observers can conclude the same information. In this sense meaning comes out of measurement and hopefully refers to reality. It is not the authors' intention to deal further with the issue of social reality inasmuch as complex philosophical issues are involved. It is sufficient to say here that reality centers some place close to the notion of agreement among many observers. It is sufficient to say that if a phenomenon exists such as client problems then it can be measured in one way or another.

43

In very concrete terms measurement links the observation of phenomena with the real world. These phenomena are called "concepts" which are called variables in the language of research. When concepts are specified into detailed parts one can assign numeric values to these elements or parts and an instrument for measuring emerges.

There are two basic goals to measurement: (1) to establish the substance of an attribute, and (2) to qualify that attribute (Edgar and Billingsley, 1974). As has been said, measurement must reflect reality and observation of real experience is the primary method of data gathering, and monitoring simply means looking systematically at some phenomenon (an emotion, behavior, etc.) over a period of time. The important issue is the definition of the observable event, feeling, or behavior. In observing and making numerical assignment to these events, feelings, and behaviors, the question of accuracy and consistency comes into mind. These concerns are centered around two basic issues: validity and reliability. Measurements must be reliable and valid. As we have said, what is measured should correspond with what is perceived. But when is a measure reliable and valid?

Reliability

Reliability is the extent to which a measure contains or does not contain variable errors; that is, errors as a consequence of differences in observation from one time to another. When this occurs then the measure is inconsistent and faulty as a tool. To put it another way, reliability could be defined as agreement and accuracy of observations and measurements; that is, they can be checked by having independent raters observe and keep records of the same target problem and compare "interobserver" rater reliability (Howe, 1974).

How can we insure the reliability of a measure? It is difficult to achieve but there are numerous approaches to the difficulty. One of the easiest things to do is to pre-test the instrument before using it with a client. Moreover, if the data collection schedule is made up of "countables"; that is, if you can count a phenomenon, then it has some validity and reliability. At least you are on your way to some minimal level of reliability. If the observer doing

the monitoring is given some training in the use of the
instruments as well as in observing, this, too, will
give considerably more reliability to your measures.
Obviously, when hard data variables are included in the
data collection schedule, variables such as day of the
week, time of the day, type of activity, higher reliability can be expected.

When doing single case studies not only does one
have to be concerned with instrument (tool) reliability
but also observer reliability. Instruments can be
tested and retested to determine consistence but observers are more difficult to control. The most pre-
ferred approach to this problem is inter-observer
reliability. Inter-observer reliability is probably
the best method of achieving reliability. This means
having two observers observing the same behavior; however, it is expensive and difficult to find a second
observer. It is equally difficult to simply find a
subject that is sufficiently controlled to actually
observe unless some institutional situation exists.

Reliability in Self-Monitoring

Because there is a great deal of self-report and
self-monitoring in doing single case studies, many
researchers discount the value of any single case work.
There are problems with self-observation but they can
be overcome if, for example, self-monitoring devices
such as watches, mini counters, diary of behavior,
portable timer, tape recorder, charts for recording
frequencies of events are employed in the data gathering process. Certain types of self-monitoring measures
can be helpful in controlling variability. They are as
follows:

a. Countables--they are easy to observe, or
actuarial frequency measures. They are discrete, need-
ing little or no judgement by the respondent.

b. All or none--measures, i.e., "you did YES or
did not NO," this measure is good for discrete data.
Did something occur or not? It is uncomplicated and
clear.

c. Recording emotion, feeling, attitude, or mood
is more complicated and requires breaking these measures down by intensity of feeling, strength of a feeling, quality of feeling such as feeling good, feeling

bad. Also, what attributes go into these feelings that make you feel good or bad? Reliability is still not good and it is difficult to check on for those kinds of variables. The best procedure to deal with this would be to train oneself as an observer. One does this all the time in the doctor's office when one is asked to report symptoms.

The accuracy of self-monitoring can be greatly improved by making use of charts, schedules, devices of one kind or another. Outside instruments provide guides to greater accuracy and reliability when carefully used by respondents. Sometimes one can have the observer record data that can be compared with the subject (client) who is under study. Watch an event and see if both observers see the same thing, as when family members are in the counselor's office setting. Have a standard recording system so data will be subject to the same interpretation when being analyzed. All of these suggestions may not be available for implementation but certainly some are inexpensive and easily applied to single case problems.

Reactivity in Self-Monitoring

Reactivity is a form of invalidity and can weaken a reliable set of instruments. When clients are asked to monitor some aspect of their behavior which is related to a problem they wish to eliminate there is likely to be a high degree of motivation to reduce the negative effects of that problem. This phenomenon is called reactivity. That is, the client is effecting the outcome he or she is monitoring. To put another way, whenever the client is involved with the collection of data regarding his or her own problem, that awareness is likely to change his or her behavior by the act of simply measuring the behavior. Fortunately, this phenomena is short-lived. However, the researcher may wish to not only control reactivity but want to use it for clinically positive reasons. Bloom and Fisher (1982) have listed a series of ways to increase reactivity as well as decrease it. Here are a few suggested ways:

Increasing Reactivity

1. Make clear value statements about the desirability of change.

2. Have the client self-monitor positive (or desirable) behaviors.

3. Set specific goals.

4. Give feedback on performance to your client.

5. Tell the client prior to intervention that his or her behaviors will or should change.

6. Focus on nonverbal behavior.

7. Have the client record prior to engaging in a target behavior.

8. Focus on only one behavior.

9. Use a very obtrusive or intrusive recording device.

10. Record on an intermittent basis or summarize at the end of the day.

Decreasing Reactivity

1. Have the client self-monitor negative (or undesirable) behaviors.

2. Focus on verbal behavior.

3. Record after the target behavior has occurred.

4. Use an unobtrusive measure.

5. Focus on more than one behavior.

6. Record on a continuous basis.

7. Wait for baseline data to be stable before starting intervention.

8. Give specific instructions to the client to try to minimize reactivity.

Validity

Validity refers to the extent of correspondence between the measurement of a variable and the intended meaning of that variable. In other words, a valid

47

measurement device is one which measures what we think it is supposed to measure. To the extent that it does just that, the instrument may be considered an effective measurement device. Also, it must be said that both issues, reliability and validity, are not separate but are linked in at least a general kind of way. That is, the truth of a measure (another definition of validity) is to some extent dependent upon its reliability. If a measurement device is inconsistently a fear of open spaces one begins to wonder if it is measuring fear let alone fear of anything. One can conclude that if a measure has high validity then its reliability is going to be relatively good, but that does not mean that the researcher should ignore the problems of reliability all together.

There are basically three kinds of validity. They are content validity, empirical validity and construct validity. Content validity refers to measures of two types: "face validity," where a number of different individuals or panel of judges agree that a measure means the same thing. The second type is sampling validity. This refers to scale items measuring a phenomenon that have been taken from a large pool of items dealing with the phenomenon in question.

Empirical validity refers to the relationship between the instrument device and the measured outcome as a consequence of using the instrument. This kind of validity is based on real experience with the tool. This kind of validity is sometimes referred to as predictive validity; that is, when one can accurately predict an outcome validity exists.

Construct validity is based on theoretical reasoning; that is, the instrument device measures a target problem which is theoretically related to other factors. For example, fear as the primary target problem is correlated with depression and loneliness. If the client suffers from loneliness or depression as well as fear then one can be assured that the instrument is measuring fear as it is an integral part of a complex of problems.

Hopefully, the practitioner will have the opportunity to select useful scales or items for monitoring purposes from previously tested scales or schedules. But even if the measures (scales, ratings, rankings, and indices) the counselor and client decide to monitor with are their own invention, they can be modified

48

after a week or so of use. This then serves as a pre-test and is most helpful to securing some amount of validity and reliability.

Internal Validity

Internal validity can be thought of as, "to what extent did the treatment actually affect the target behavior?" Campbell and Stanley (1963) insist that internal validity is the basic minimum required in order to interpret the results. Factors affecting internal validity include: history, maturation, selection, testing and mortality. These have been discussed earlier in the chapter on design. In the group comparison approach internal validity is obtained through the use of equivalent groups and through randomization. Internal validity with single case designs is achieved through variations of a reversal design, which attempts to show a reliable control of the dependent variable by the independent variable (Edgar and Billingsley, 1974). The critical technique used in ideographic research to establish internal validity is replication or multiple phases (Edgar and Billingsley, 1974). Each successful replication of the experiment decreases the probability that chance affected the change (Sidman, 1960). One must remember that the practitioner is not measuring all the client's behavior and should try to keep the observations and measurements as simple, concise, and economical as possible so that replication is easily carried out. A very extensive data collection done on a day-to-day basis through lengthy replication can be extremely laborious (Howe, 1974). One should collect as many dependent variables as possible, yet it may be expensive to do so (15 to 20 may be too large but 4 to 5, 10 to 12 may be sufficient). This should be thought out carefully.

Instrumentation (Scaling Variables)

In this section we wish to briefly discuss some common kinds of scales and measures. Most instruments used in research work are single questions and in some cases a single scale is used as instrument and schedule. It should be remembered from earlier discussion that a schedule contains one or more instruments. Most schedules do indeed contain several instruments. In this section we will examine single instruments as illustrated in Scale 1, 2, 3, and 4. Logs 1 and 2 are special cases that illustrate a special type of measure.

One series of instruments is based on a single set of numeric values which may run 1 to 5, or 1 to 7, or 0 to 10 as seen in Scales 1, 2, and 3. In Scale 1 the two extreme ends of the scale are "anchored" with explicit descriptions of what those points of intensity mean. The respondent can then make a judgement as to the point at or between the extremes he or she falls in attitude or experience. In Scale 2 a self-anchoring instrument is made up of a five point scale of intensity. In this example all five points have been separately defined for the respondent. Normally, these descriptors are not included on the final data collection schedule, yet the respondent or monitor will train her or himself in the meaning of each point on the scale before proceeding with the monitor process. Scale 3 is a seven point instrument where each of the

Scale 1.

ANXIETY SCALE WITH SUBJECTIVE ANCHORING POINTS

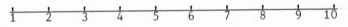

Anchoring of Zero

Feeling of total
relaxation such as
that which is felt
as I lay leisurely
on a sunny beach
after an exhiler-
ating swim.

Anchoring of Ten

Feeling of tension
such as that felt
when I have an exam
for which I have
not yet prepared
and a paper due
which is not yet
completed.

seven points have been defined for the monitor. This arrangement is probably best because little is left to the imagination of the respondent. This process of defining points on an interval scale increases relia- bility and reduces individual respondent judgement. It is therefore suggested that when scales of this kind are used each point on that scale should be defined first before extensive use is made of it. That is done by first defining the two extremes and then developing gradations of feeling in between the extremes. This

50

Scale 2.

A Self Anchoring Scale

GENERAL ATTITUDINAL (MOOD) SCALE

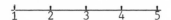

1. Feel exhausted physically, moody and irritable, can't wait until the day is over.

2. Feel tired but not totally drained, as #1. Things could be a lot better but not feeling irritable.

3. General mood is "so-so," able to press on during the day although not getting as much sleep as desired.

4. Physically rested. Generally feel that things are going all right for me.

5. Feel physically strong, adequate sleep, good general physical condition. Able to accomplish many activities and feel strong. Things are going well.

Scale 3.

SCALE FOR MONITORING SLEEP

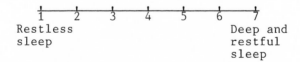

Restless   Deep and
sleep   restful
                  sleep

1. Uneasy and unquiet sleep, awakening several times during the night before. Unable to fall asleep again. Feeling headache, need medication.

2. Unpeaceful sleep. Unable to fall asleep at moment to go to bed, late

51

      in the evening. Checking the
clock several times. Needed
medication for a headache.

3.   Superficial sleep, but awakening
more than three times and having
nightmares. Difficulty in falling
asleep but rapid feeling of com-
fort.

4.   Superficial sleep, awakening
several times but falling asleep
rapidly. Some difficulty at
moment to go to bed.

5.   Superficial sleep, awakening only
one time, and any difficulty
at moment to go to bed.

6.   Quiet sleep but not intense,
slight awakes at night but not
totally awakened. Any difficulty
in falling asleep.

7.   Intense and continuous heavy sleep
seven hours the night before.
Peaceful sleep. Fall asleep
rapidly.

process is akin to what every researcher does when
developing a questionnaire or schedule, i.e., setting
up variables and defining the categories of those variables.

When doing single case research the respondent is
gathering data on a rather frequent basis; that is,
more than once a day, once each day, or every two or
three days. Because the monitor is using the same instrument over and over again and doing so frequently,
the schedule needs to be relatively short, as will be
seen in the next section of this chapter. Long schedules; that is, any set of instruments of over one 8½ x
11 page is laborious and only encourages non-compliance
on the part of the monitor. However, there are times
when a special scale is needed to get at a particular
problem and a longer instrument should be used.

Scale 4 is such an example of a multiple item
scale. Up to this point Scales 1, 2, and 3 are single

dimensional and therefore brief and uncomplicated. Scale 4, which measures "coping" with one's job, is made up of 20 items which must be filled out once for each unit of observation. It is also possible to randomly select ten items from this kind of scale and thereby reduce the amount of effort to complete the scale. It should be remembered that the value of a longer scale such as this is that it has high reliability. Of course, researchers should always try to make use of scales that have already been tested or used by other practitioners or researchers.

Finally, there are other kinds of tools that are of great value to the monitoring process; namely, logs or journals that are maintained by the respondent-client. The specific value of these logs or journals is that they serve to validate the data being gathered in the usual monitoring process previously described. Bloom and Fisher (1982) present in their book a series of logs. One type of log is a record of the time an important event has occurred and the client's reaction to that event. This same kind of "measure" has been built into schedule 3 and 6, as presented in the next section on schedule formats. The second type is like the first, only it provides much more detail about events and the occurrence of critical instants. When this kind of information is gathered, it, along with the usual monitoring data, can be plotted on graphs and serve as the basis of significant discussion between the client and practitioner.

Scale 4.

THE COPING CHECKLIST

The Coping Checklist is designed to provide a very rough and superficial approximation of how well you are now coping with your job in comparison with the idealized model.

COPING CHECKLIST

To what extent does each of the following fit as a description of you? (Circle one number in each line across.)

		Very true	Quite true	Some-what true	Not very true	Not at all true
1.	I "roll with the punches" when problems come up.	1	2	3	4	5
2.	I spend almost all of my time thinking about my work.	5	4	3	2	1
3.	I treat other people as individuals and care about their feelings and opinions.	1	2	3	4	5
4.	I recognize and accept my own limitations and assets.	1	2	3	4	5
5.	There are quite a few people I could describe as "good friends."	1	2	3	4	5
6.	I enjoy using my skills and abilities both on and off the job.	1	2	3	4	5
7.	I get bored easily.	5	4	3	2	1
8.	I enjoy meeting and talking with people who have different ways of thinking about the world.	1	2	3	4	5
9.	Often in my job I "bite off more than I can chew."	5	4	3	2	1
10.	I'm usually very active on weekends with projects or recreation.	1	2	3	4	5
11.	I prefer working with people who are					

		Very true	Quite true	Some-what true	Not very true	Not at all true
	very much like myself.	5	4	3	2	1
12.	I work primarily because I have to survive, and not necessarily because I enjoy what I do.	5	4	3	2	1
13.	I believe I have a realistic picture of my personal strengths and weaknesses.	1	2	3	4	5
14.	Often I get into arguments with people who don't think my way.	5	4	3	2	1
15.	Often I have trouble getting much done on my job.	5	4	3	2	1
16.	I'm interested in a lot of different topics.	1	2	3	4	5
17.	I get upset when things don't go my way.	5	4	3	2	1
18.	Often I'm not sure how I stand on a controversial topic.	5	4	3	2	1
19.	I'm usually able to find a way around anything which blocks me from an important goal.	1	2	3	4	5
20.	I often disagree with my boss or others at work.	5	4	3	2	1

Scoring Directions

Add together the numbers you circled for the four questions contained in each of the five coping scales.

Coping scale	Add together your responses to these questions	Your score (write in)
Knows self	4, 9, 13, 18	_____
Many interests	2, 5, 7, 16	_____
Variety of reactions	1, 11, 17, 19	_____
Accepts other's values	3, 8, 14, 20	_____
Active and productive	6, 10, 12, 15	_____

Then, add the five scores together for your overall total score: _____

Scores on each of the five areas can vary between 5 and 20. Scores of 12 or above perhaps suggest that it might be useful to direct more attention to the area.

The overall total score can range between 20 and 100. Scores of 60 or more may suggest some general difficulty in coping on the dimensions covered.

The Data Collection Schedule Format

When practitioners are at work, they, like most everyone else, has a routine that is filled with more than enough activity. It is the belief of the authors that the single case study used in conjunction with counseling should be done rigorously and with care, but at the same time should fit the worker's and client's situation. That is, how complicated can the study be? How much time can the worker give to the instructing of the client in the use of data gathering? We feel the use of single case is integral to the treatment process but many workers need to be convinced. The following series of examples of data schedules are suggestions only and can be greatly modified to fit the client-practitioner situation. At the extreme, even simple monitoring <u>without</u> an instrument or schedule will be of value to the client-practitioner relationship.

The data collection schedule should be designed to fit the work schedule and work pattern of the practitioner and client. The schedule should be:

1. Small in size, if possible, on half sheet of paper (5 x 8), or even a smaller pad.

2. Each schedule should be a single sheet that can be moved about separately.

3. If necessary, one should devise it in such a way as to make it convenient to carry about.

4. Items should be set up for convenience, each item or variable with categories with spaces for easy recording or checking.

5. Designing with care will mean easier manipulation of data when processing and graphing begins.

Furthermore, a behavioral code should be observed when designing the schedule. A behavioral code is a definition of <u>when</u>, <u>what</u>, <u>where</u> and <u>how</u> something is observed. This means you should specify these conditions for each variable on your data collection schedule. They include the following:

a. Duration of a behavior

b. The number of times a behavior occurs

c. Day of week

d. Phase

e. Schedule number

Schedules numbered 1 through 6 are presented in the following pages. These have all been taken from actual single case studies. The designs are all in many respects different in order to give the reader a clearer idea of the range of possible designs based on different purposes. It should be noted that an asterisk denotes primary target problems being monitored. Also, when one examines each of these it will be noted that they all include the item "phase." If there are variations in the number and type of phase this can be

designed into the schedule to meet the needs of the
specific problem studied. Schedule number is also included on all six in order that sequence be maintained
for the time when analysis begins. Day of the week is
another item common to all schedules inasmuch as behavior is to a great extent determined by the time of the
week such as "weekend" and "week day." Finally, the
nature of problems shown here is only illustrative, for
the practitioner will naturally let the focus be on the
needs and problems of the client.

Schedule 1.

A STUDY OF CIGARETTE SMOKING REDUCTION

1. Schedule Number: _____

2. Day of the Week: Sat __ Sun __ Mon __ Tues __
   Wed __ Thurs __ Fri __

3. Number of Cigarettes in Pack (Morning): _____

4. Quality of Sleep: Excellent 1 __ 2 __ 3 __
   4 __ 5 __ Very poor

5. Minutes to Run Half-Mile: _____

6. Breathing Effort: None 1 __ 2 __ 3 __ 4 __
   5 __ A great deal

7. Degree of Fatigue (5-6 pm): None 1 __ 2 __ 3 __
   4 __ 5 __ A great deal

*8. Number of Cigarettes Smoked During the Day: _____

9. Phase: Baseline _____ Intervention _____
   Withdrawal _____

Schedule 2.

MONITORING MARITAL CONFLICTS

1. Schedule Number: _____

2. Day of the Week: Sat __ Sun __ Mon __ Tues __
   Wed __ Thurs __ Fri __

*3. Number of times I felt anger for spouse: _____

*4. Number of times I quarrelled with spouse: _____

*5. Number of times I expressed hostility (anger) at
   children: _____

6. Did you feel depressed during the day? Very 1 __
   2 __ 3 __ 4 __ 5 __ 6 __ 7 __ Not at all

7. Feelings of tightness, rigidity, or tenseness in
   body? ☐ Extreme tenseness ☐ Uncomfortable
   tenseness ☐ Moderate tenseness ☐ Slight
   tenseness ☐ No tenseness

8. General description of quality of sleep experienced during nighttime hours: ☐ Very good
   ☐ Good ☐ Average ☐ Poor ☐ Very poor

9. Phase: Baseline _____ Intervention _____
   Withdrawal _____

Schedule 3.

SELF-MONITORING DESIGN: A STUDY OF TEASING BEHAVIOR

1. Schedule Number: _____
2. Day of the Week: Sat __ Sun __ Mon __ Tues __
   Wed __   Thurs __   Fri __
3. Phase: Baseline _____ Intervention _____
   Withdrawal _____
4. Time of Day when Occurrences of "Teasing" Behavior were noted: Morning _____ Afternoon _____
   Evening _____
*5. Number of Occurrences of "Teasing" Behavior:
   0 __ 1 __ 2 __ 3 __ 4 __ 5 __ 6 __ 7 __
*6. Number of Times "Teasing" Behavior was considered:
   0 __ 1 __ 2 __ 3 __ 4 __ 5 __ 6 __ 7 __
7. Type of Activity (Being Involved in) at Time of
   Occurrence of "Teasing" Behavior: Studying __
   Housework __ Playing __ Discussion __ Watching
   TV __ Riding in Auto __ Discussion at Bedtime __
   Other _____

Schedule 4.

MONITORING NECK AND SHOULDER DISCOMFORT

1. Schedule Number: _____

2. Day of the Week: Sat __ Sun __ Mon __ Tues __
   Wed __ Thurs __ Fri __

3. Overall Life Satisfaction: Worst 1 2 3 4 5
   6 7 Best possible

4. Number of Times Quarrelled with Wife: Worst 1 2
   3 4 5 6 7 Best possible

*5. Rating of Discomfort: None 1 Barely notice it 2
   Notice it 3 Hurts a little 4 Hurts moderately 5
   Hurts a lot 6 Trouble turning head 7

6. Affects on Activity after Noticing Discomfort:
   No difference 1 Hardly any 2 Some 3 Moderate 4
   Fair amount 5 A lot 6 Incapacitating 7

7. Number of Times Focused on Discomfort: 1 2 3
   4 5 6 7

8. Time of Relaxation Training (Number of Minutes):

   _____

9. Minutes Stretching: 0 5 10 15 20 25 30 35

10. Phase: Baseline _____ Intervention _____
    Withdrawal _____

Schedule 5.

```
MONITORING ASSERTIVE BEHAVIOR

 1. Schedule Number:  _____
 2. Day of the Week:  Sat __  Sun __  Mon __  Tues __
    Wed __   Thurs __  Fri __
*3. Count the Number of Times Each Day that You are
    Compliant ("Giving In"):  _____
*4. Number of Times You Expressed Disagreement With
    Others:  _____
*5. Number of Times You Act Out Disagreement:  _____
*6. Number of Times You Say "No" Today:  _____
 7. Number of Times I Felt Anger Physically:  1  2  3
    4  5  6  7  ____
 8. How I Feel About Myself Today:  Good 1  2  3  4
    5  6  7 Bad  ____
 9. Experimental Phase:  Baseline _____  Treat-
    ment _____  Withdrawal _____
10. Treatment Variable:  _____
```

Schedule 6.

A STUDY OF THE EFFECT OF EXERCISE
ON PERSONAL HABITS AND HEALTH

1. Schedule Number: _____

2. Day of the Week: Sat __ Sun __ Mon __ Tues __
   Wed __ Thurs __ Fri __

3. Special Events: _____

*4. Number of Cigarettes Smoked: _____

*5. Weight before Bedtime: _____

*6. General Attitude Rating (Last Two Hours of Work
   or 4-6 pm): Very tired 1 2 3 4 5 6 7 Very
   vigorous

*7. Relaxation Rating (6 pm): Very relaxed 1   2   3
   4   5   6   7 Very tense

8. Hours of Sleep: _____

9. Phase: Baseline _____ Treatment 1 _____
   Treatment 2 _____

CHAPTER 5

COLLECTING AND DISPLAYING DATA

Now that the data collection schedule has been designed with all the necessary instruments included, the collection of data can begin. The data collection process for survey research is done by personal interview, agency or program records, from groups gathered together, or mailed questionnaires. For traditional experimental work data are collected at some point before the application of an intervention and then sometime after it has been removed. In any event, the researcher is taking and recording the data from a respondent or the respondent is responding to a data collection schedule provided by the researcher. In the collection of data in single case research the data are collected by the researcher who is also the respondent, in other words, self report or else it is collected by a researcher (observer) observing another person, the respondent. In most clinical situations it is the client who has been trained by the practitioner who collects the data from her or himself.

Collecting Single Case Data

Most single case designs use direct observational (observation of self) data which result in the collection of continuous data. The advantages of continuous data, as compared to pre/post or one time only data, are numerous. Specifically, continuous data provide many points which eliminate the drastic effects of one or two highly variable points; exact relationships may be demonstrated between the dependent and independent variables over time (latency effects); and most important, change in the dependent variable is demonstrated across time (Edgar and Billingsley, 1974). Obviously, each point in time is what we call a data point, which provides the basis of trends and patterns for the single case being studied.

The unit of time over which the data are collected has to be decided before the establishment of the baseline. It can be: one measurement a day, twice daily, once a week, once every hour, etc. This decision will be based on: (1) the length of time necessary for the target behavior to occur, and (2) the amount of change one can anticipate from one point of observation to

another. One can solve this problem by taking a TIME
SWEEP. That is, a random time sample which is the pre/
selection of sample moments. When the sample moment
comes up, then make the observation. Hopefully, the
unit of time will include target behavior or activity
or will be observed frequently enough to catch the target behavior. If the unit is too broad, there will be
too much "noise." "Noise" refers to influences other
than the intended intervention. Probably the most
common unit of observation is the single day.

Establishing a baseline requires collecting data
basically for stability. One must always establish a
baseline of observations first. It is best to accumulate at least 10 points of observation. This number is
suggested because stability of measurement pattern is
likely with that number. In some situations you may
need fewer points of observation. If one is doing self-
monitoring it is necessary to establish a steady state
before intervention. This is especially important because self-monitoring produces a good deal of variability (reactivity) in the beginning phases of a single
case study. The number of data points needed in this
case may be determined pragmatically by the researcher
respondent. When the researcher is observing another
person, a "steady state" may be established more quickly and thereby requiring fewer data points.

If the practitioner is to ask the client to parti-
cipate in the collection of data about her or himself
then the practitioner may have to encourage the client
to do so. The client with normal intelligence can do
self-monitoring if carefully and properly instructed in
the use of the data collection schedule with its various
instruments. The writers' experience is that clients
can do it if they have agreed and participated in the
planning of the project from the beginning. When the
client returns for counseling after the first week or
so of self-monitoring, the practitioner can make any
corrections necessary for more accurate and precise
data gathering. Obviously one should encourage through
praising the efforts of the client up to that point.
Again, experience with clients doing single case studies shows that clients can do this and do it well with
adequate instruction. Other positive things happen to
the client when self-monitoring takes place. That is,
positive things in terms of the counseling aspects of
the client-worker relationship. Clients see the problem more clearly and have a strong sense of control of
the counseling process.

Recording Data

The actual recording of information on the data collection schedule should occur at the end of each unit of observation (time sweep). For example, if the unit of observation is defined as a single day, during which activity and behavior is occurring, then the recording should occur at the end of the day. If the target behavior occurs at different times, then it is best to record at or immediately after the behavior has happened. The event or behavior should be observed and recorded (documented) as closely as possible to the occurrence of the events. The recording of observations should be as simple and unobtrusive as possible. The routine of work and leisure should be undisturbed by the observing and recording process. This can be greatly aided if all categories to all items (instruments) have been worked out and printed on the schedule before the data collection process begins. This way, quick and easy checking is possible without disrupting one's routine.

If client logs or journals are used in addition to the regular monitoring of the target problem, they can be used for observing the special events and circumstances surrounding the occurrence of the problem or behavior in question. These logs prepared by the client can be used with great effectiveness in conjunction with scales and ratings used in the day-to-day monitoring process.

The Management and Processing of Data

As the data are being collected, it is important to re-examine each schedule for completeness and accuracy at the end of each time sweep. The client should be reminded to be accurate and complete a schedule for each time sweep unit. It is probably best to remind the client to store all data schedules in a safe place until the study is complete or until the next counseling session when the client should be encouraged to bring with her or him the data collected since the last counseling session. At that point, the data can be examined, graphed and become the basis for discussion. But it is important not to examine the data during the collection process because one is subject to bias in one direction or another. This is especially true in the early (baseline) phase. After the process is under way, collecting becomes routine and a true pattern can emerge. If one is tempted to examine the data it should be done either at the end of a phase or at counseling sessions as mentioned above.

When a week or a phase of data has been accumulated the data needs to be prepared for display. If the data are to be computerized then it will be necessary to code each schedule in accordance with those procedures of an appropriate computer language. At this point, we will not go into this procedure here but will in later chapters. As more and more agencies acquire computer equipment and the technical skill to use such equipment, procedures for transferring data into computer routines will become common and will speed up analysis of single case data. With such speed up, this information will become even more valuable to the client and practitioner.

Displaying Data

One might argue that the displaying of one's data is the first step in the process of data analysis. That is true to a certain extent, but for now let us be satisfied with getting a chance to examine the data in the more traditional manner, namely <u>tabulation and graphic presentation</u>. This phase of the single case study is very valuable because we are able to make comparisons using frequencies and mean (average) values which are common to most educated and even less educated persons.

Data should be processed and displayed because this serves to help bring the counselors' practice activities under the control of the results (Thomas, 1975). Tables, bar charts, cumulative frequency curves, histograms, line graphs, are all beneficial and should be utilized according to what best represents the data. Most importantly, the data should be clear and concise so that one who is not familiar with the project will understand the data displayed.

There are a number of different ways to display one's data. The two ways discussed here are frequency tabulation and line graphs. One could use bar charts, pie charts, pictorials, and cumulative frequency curves. Researchers in most single case projects hand tabulate their observations, however, as indicated earlier, a growing number of projects will be committed to computer analysis. Since you will be dealing with a small

68

number of observations, the processing is relatively simple. The procedure for tabulation is not complicated. It is referred to as "sort, count, and record" and is done by hand. The major factor upon which one should sort, count and record is "phase." You may first sort out by phase and then by each of the dependent variables. Sorting by phase refers to (A) Baseline, (B) Intervention, and (A) Withdrawal if such a phase is included as a part of the project.

An example of the sort, count and record process is illustrated in Tables 1, 2, and 3. It will be noted that the schedules for the baseline phase have been sorted out into the categories of the first ten observations as to how fearful the client was at that time. Then the same was done for intervention and withdrawal. It will then be noted that a mean value has been computed for each of the three phases as that now clear comparisons can be made between and among phases.

Table 1.

FREQUENCY OF TARGET BEHAVIOR:
FEAR OF HEIGHT, BY PHASE WITH MEAN VALUES

	PHASES		
Observations	Baseline	Intervention	Withdrawal
1	2	3	2
2	2	4	3
3	4	4	3
4	5	6	3
5	4	5	3
6	2	4	2
7	2	4	2
8	3	5	2
9	3	5	3
10	4	6	3
	$\overline{X}$=3.1	$\overline{X}$=4.6	$\overline{X}$=2.6

Table 2 is a somewhat different tabulation arrangement. This is a summary table of mean values taken from tables such as in Table 1. Here again, comparisons

Table 2.

MEAN VALUES FOR PRIMARY AND OTHER VARIABLES BY PHASE

Other depen-dent variables	PHASES		
	Baseline	Intervention	Withdrawal
Amount of alcohol	2.5	1.5	2.8
Hours drinking	3.8	2.1	4.1
Mood during	4.2	3.8	4.8
Mood next day	5.7	3.5	6.1

Table 3.

FREQUENCY OF SMOKING CIGARETTES FOR
SUB-SECTIONS OF THE DAY BY PHASE

Time of Day	PHASE		
	Baseline	Intervention	Withdrawal
Morning	7	3	8
Afternoon	8	5	9
Evening	14	8	17
Daily Total	29	16	34

can be made between and among phases on several different variables related to the primary target problem
(excessive drinking in this case). One can see, for
example, that the amount of alcohol consumed, duration
of the consumption, mood during and mood the following
day were all lower in numerical value for the intervention phase compared to either the baseline or withdrawal phase.

Table 3 shows the client and counselor the frequency of cigarette smoking by phase of the study but also by sub-section of the day which is the unit of observation. Here again it is possible to compare not only phase to phase, but time of day by phase. This kind of display makes it possible to pinpoint what particular time of the day is the client smoking the most or least.

Table 4 displays another kind of data by phase. Here one can see that special kinds of events which are not routinely happening everyday but only occasionally can be grouped into phases and compared as to their frequency during each phase of the project. Again it is possible to see the kinds of activities that are occurring most often and least often for the client. The total at the bottom of the table gives the client and counselor an overall frequency count of activity by phase.

Table 4.

FREQUENCY OF NON-SCALED VARIABLES
BY PHASE (RELAXATION EVENTS)

Variables	PHASES		
	Baseline	Intervention	Withdrawal
Dining out	2	2	3
Movies	1	1	1
Parties	1	1	1
TV watching	5	4	5
Sports	1	1	1
Running	3	5	1
Yoga	1	5	2
Total	14	19	14

Unusual events can be organized this way to see patterns of gross changes.

71

CHAPTER 6

METHODS OF DATA ANALYSIS

Introduction

Once the collection of data is completed, the single subject project will take a new direction. Although each phase of the single case design is important, it is through the analysis of the data that the information sought will emerge. The interdependence between measurement and instrumentation is an important one. If dependent or target behavior variables and independent or intervention variables were not operationalized carefully, the data analysis will not yield useful information. In other words, the clarity of the instruments will be reflected in the analysis of data.

It is important not to actually use analytical methods until the entire monitoring phase of the project is over. Preliminary tabulation and preparation of graphs may begin somewhat sooner; however, as noted in the previous chapter, only at the end of a phase. If the practitioner has done the tabulating this rule does not have to be so rigidly applied; however, practitioners should be careful not to disrupt the monitoring and only ask for the data at logical stopping points, like phase changes.

Allowing enough time to discuss the data after it has been tabulated and graphed with the client is an important consideration practitioners must consider in terms of the total number of contacts the client will have with the agency. Here, these decisions depend on how involved and aware the client is of the entire single case project. Some practitioners may only involve the client in the monitoring, or depending on the client and the situation the client may have a vested interest in understanding the modes of analysis. The important point is that the practitioner adapts the single case project to her or his individual professional style and the client. The practitioner may want to devote one session to a discussion of the results after she or he more carefully analyzes the data, and makes some notes. Since in most cases the clients will be doing monitoring, they will have some interest in the data, at least in discussing the simple graphic and tabular displays.

73

Although the designated single case project may be over, certainly treatment or client sessions may not be. Many practitioners encourage the client to continue the monitoring, perhaps another withdrawal phase after the initial design, ABA or ABAB (or whatever design is utilized) is over. Many clients will have incorporated the monitoring into their lives and it may be helpful for many reasons to have them continue monitoring, even if it's on a limited basis. This may be valuable if the practitioner wants to see more data after the first round of analysis.

As the variability of single system designs has been expressed in Chapter 1, again, there is not one mode of analysis for this type of data, but many methods; at least eight different methods have been utilized: (1) Experiential Analysis, (2) Visual Inspection Techniques, (3) Split Middle Method of Trend Estimation, (4) Celeration Line or Semiaverage Method, (5) Relative Frequency Technique, (6) Two Standard Deviation Technique, (7) The T-Test, and (8) The Analysis of Variance. In this chapter we shall discuss the first three methods and in Chapter 7 the statistical methods will be treated.

Experiential Analysis

Experiential analysis refers to the qualitative judgements of the clinician-researcher and the client. This method is used by all practitioners without any reference to a single system design. It is basically clinical judgements within a single case framework; one is making reference to the experience of monitoring and worker and client perceptions of change without formal reference to graphs and tables.

Workers often are required to document all client contact and this documentation may include some sort of social history or clinical record of client progress. The worker can use her notes recorded about the client during baseline and compare to her notes taken when the intervention was added in the client's life. Workers often can note changes in their clients independent of the actual data collected.

The client, in addition, may be able to testify to changes regarding behavior or attitudes toward behavior. If the client has kept a diary, journal or log, this may provide valuable information. This type of data may be considered unobtrusive, especially if it has been collected independent of the monitoring effort.

In cases where the only instruments used were logs or journals, qualitative analysis may be the only type of analysis performed. In these cases more clinical judgement will be applied as to how to interpret what the client is recording. The worker may look for key behavior or attitude changes, or any relevant difference in the clients which may be due to the intervention. Many of the psychoanalytic verbal anxiety measures involve a client recording any thought, in the form of free association. The clinician then codes the data according to a predetermined scheme reflecting psychoanalytic categories of anxiety.

Practitioners frequently make reference to experiential analysis as "social validation." That is, not only does the worker make observations based on experience with the client, but the client, as well, can make assessments about his or her sense of change. In addition to that material, significant others can provide relevant comments regarding the client's presumed progress and change in attitude, mood and behavior.

Most likely, experiential analysis is inherent to the therapeutic process and within single systems studies, the utility of experiential analysis is as an accompaniment to the more refined and precise measures. Its power is often as an aid to interpreting visual and statistical results, especially in unclear or borderline situations, where results are almost significant, or where a graph may not reveal some of the changes.

Visual Inspection of Raw Data Points: Graphic Presentation

Every text or article written on the subject of single case research will state with clear emphasis that the basic tool for the analysis of single case data is the graph. Graphing single case data moves one's data closer to that phase of the research referred to as analysis and interpretation. The purchase and use of graph paper is essential. Graph paper comes in a variety of sizes from very small grids to large ones. One can even make graph paper if it is carefully drawn where the grids create perfect squares large or small.

Each variable or target problem should be represented on a graph of its own so that it can be presented very clearly to client and counselor for study and discussion. In Graph 1, two factors are indicated that are always present on any single case graph, and that is time and problem. Time is always placed on the horizontal (abscissa) and the target behavior or problem on the vertical (see ABA design in Graph 1).

Graph 1.

ILLUSTRATION OF A BASIC GRAPH
REPRESENTING BEHAVIOR BY TIME

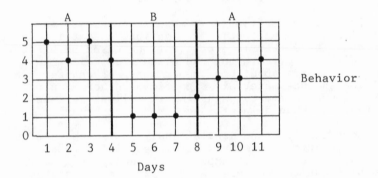

Graphing is done by first examining the measure of the first day of the project and recording that measure on the vertical line representing the first day. If it is a "3" then a dot is placed at the intersection of day one and behavior measure 3. The researcher turns to the second day and finds the value of the measured behavior and locates the dot on the second vertical line and the horizontal line. This procedure is continued until all data points have been plotted.

The data when collected for one phase can be plotted immediately and then discussed by client and counselor. One can wait until all data are collected for all phases. Each observation for each variable for one day is a data point. All data points should be plotted on the graph. Plotting the following data--3,5,4,7,2,5,6,4,9--one can then connect each dot (data point) with a straight line. This gives a visual representation of the data through time. All graphs

should have graphed squares of the same dimension. All
phases should be graphed on one page. Graphing with
grids makes it possible to visually make systematic and
proportional judgements that are fairly accurate. The
eye is the analyzer and the graph a tool to aid in the
analysis. After plotting your data, observe the trend.
At this point, analysis begins.

Unlike many other modes of analysis, which rely
entirely on mathematical models and equations, single
case research has a long history of utilizing a visual
model for analysis. The alienation often produced by
just looking at "numbers" is not a concern with analysis of single case data. Here the analysis is much more
holistic and integrated. Certainly numerical values
are utilized, but they are always connected to their
context which is most likely a graph or chart. Even
when statistics are discussed, it is always in conjunction with a visual model. Thus the researchers,
both client and counselor, are brought much closer to
the data.

The case for visual inspection is not only rein-
forced by statisticians, but by the objective sought
after by the practitioner. The practitioner usually
is criterion-oriented and requires visual and behavioral proof that a particular intervention is significant. The clinical requirement for "significant" may
be an observable level of behavioral change adequate to
function in certain social situations. As Kazdin notes
(1976: 267), statistical evidence stamped "significant"
may indicate a change that would fall far short of the
requirements of the social service practitioner. This
issue shall be more fully discussed in Chapter 7.

"Eyeballing" the data is the first and most basic
form of visual inspection. The term "eyeballing" is
used to denote that the human eye is an important
analytic tool. The eye will see a series of dots as a
gestalt or whole picture. The client and the practitioner may view the graphed data points from a series
of angles and can note directions, plateaus, regres-
sions, or inconsistencies. Before any more sophisticated methods are used, all charts and graphs should
be carefully inspected and reviewed. The practitioner
should begin to gain a feel for the data by noting any
changes in means or in the shape or curve of the data
points once they have been connected on the graph.

For example, a look at Graph 2 indicates that the

77

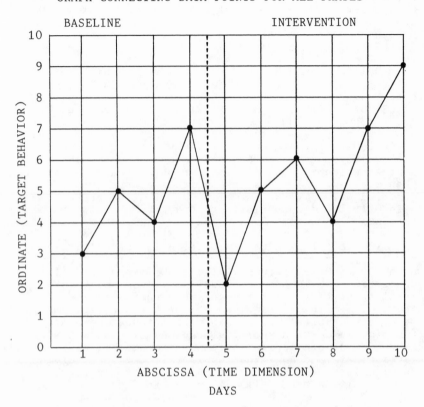

Graph 2.

GRAPH CONNECTING DATA POINTS FOR ALL PHASES

BASELINE   INTERVENTION

ORDINATE (TARGET BEHAVIOR)

ABSCISSA (TIME DIMENSION)

DAYS

data was more varied during intervention than during baseline. Certainly towards the end of intervention something unusual was happening, as the data points steadily begin to climb.

The Split Middle Method of Trend Estimation

The Split Middle Method represents a way to deter- mine trends or patterns in each phase. A celeration line is calculated from the data points (just as they are, and not connected by straight lines) on the graph. A celeration line is drawn for each phase and this line

78

will represent the typical performance for the phase. After the celeration line is drawn for each phase, the previously outlined visual inspection model can be applied. In fact, one can easily compute a rate of change within a phase and changes across phases. In addition, one can use the calculated celeration line for the baseline period as a predictor of the celeration line for the intervention period. This is a statistical approach to the visual data and will be discussed in the following chapter. Regardless if numbers will be applied to the celeration lines, they still should be drawn as they have great descriptive value in telling the client and counselor more about the data. Visually, they represent the median or most typical rate of behavior or whatever was monitored.

The steps and directions for drawing a celeration line are illustrated below. The first figure represents the final step.

Figure 20.

CELERATION LINES FOR ALL THREE PHASES

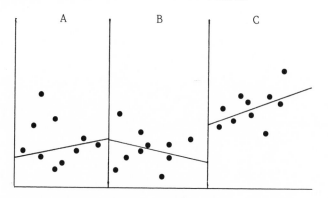

Celeration line

These are the calculated celeration lines, which represent the typical performance during a phase. Half of the data points within a phase should fall below the celeration line and half of the data points should be above the celeration line. Applying the visual inspection model one could make the interpretation that there is a linear trend or drift present in all three phases. A change in level and slope across

phases can also be seen. The trend of drift is in opposite directions and thus the drift is not across
phases.

Figure 21.

SPLIT MIDDLE TREND ESTIMATION PROCEDURES

Step 1:

Data Points for Three Phases

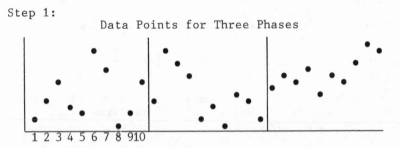

1 2 3 4 5 6 7 8 910

Data should be graphed; however, the connecting
lines need not be drawn in. If they are, be sure to
use a different color of pencil for the split middle
method.

Figure 22.

STEP 2 IN CALCULATING THE CELERATION LINE

A celeration line is drawn for each
phase; one line for phase A, one for B, and
so forth. From this point on, we will consider one phase at a time. First, divide
the first phase (A) in half by drawing a
vertical line at the median where an
equal number of data points fall on each
side or through a data point if there is
an odd number. There will be an equal
number on each side.

Figure 22, continued

Phase A Data Points

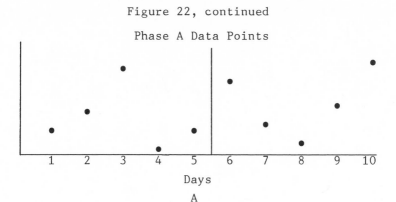

Days

A

Figure 23.

STEP 3 IN CALCULATING THE CELERATION LINE

You want to determine the median rate
of performance for the first and second halves
of the phase (phase A). There are five data
points for each half of phase A. So 3 is
the median of five points.

Now select the median point for each
half by counting over 3 data points from the
bottom of the graph toward the top data
point for the first half. Draw a line
horizontally through this point. In the
example below, the third data point is on
the same line as two other data points.
Next, draw a vertical line along at the
median point for the first half by counting
from the data point at the extreme left to
the third data point. The vertical line
will cross the horizontal line.

Now, repeat this for the second half
of phase A.

81

Figure 24.

SPLIT MIDDLE FOR HALF PHASES USING MEDIAN,
BOTH VERTICAL AND HORIZONTAL

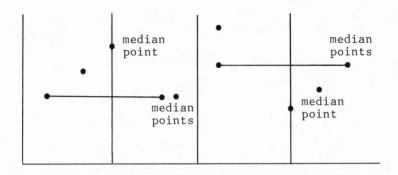

Figure 25.

FINAL CELERATION LINE FOR PHASE A

The last step is to draw a straight
line (this is the celeration line) from the
intersection of the horizontal and vertical
from the first half of phase A to the intersection of the horizontal and vertical lines
from the second half of phase A.

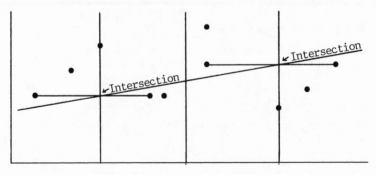

Phase A Celeration Line

Does the line split in the middle of
the data points? So that 50% are above and
50% are below the celeration lines? You may
adjust the split middle line so it equally
divides all the data points. (The line
may have to be moved but without changing
the slope.) It will be parallel to the
original line.

As you can see there are five data
points below the celeration line and five
points above it. Now repeat these steps
for each phase.

Once the celeration line is drawn for each phase,
the pattern of data will emerge. One can compute the
rate of change (slope) within a phase simply by locat-
ing where the celeration line falls on the first and
last days of the phase. This value, of course, depends
on what you are measuring, what behavior, mood, or
feeling, the graph represents. Nevertheless, at what
values is the celeration line at on the first and last
days of a phase? The ratio of change is computed by
dividing the larger value by the smaller value. Our
concept of level can be expressed as the value of the
data point of the last day within each phase.

One can evaluate changes across phases by comparing the levels and the slopes or ratio of change.
Computing a change in slope across phases can be done
by dividing the larger slope value by the smaller
slope value. If the slopes are in opposite directions
(e.g., baseline slope is accelerating and intervention
slope is decelerating), then multiply the values instead of dividing. This procedure is explained more
fully in Hersen and Barlow (1976).

The basic purpose of this method is to summarize
the data in each phase without distorting or altering
it in order to give the client and practitioner a more
clear picture of what was happening during baseline and
intervention phases. One musn't get overwhelmed with
the notions of levels and slopes. Remember the levels
and slopes represent a client's life situation and this
data should be carefully attended to.

Visual Inspection of Celeration Lines

Kazdin (1976) presents a series of visual models to demonstrate a model of visual analysis. The model presents three basic characteristics to observe for, before, during and after the intervention. The three characteristics are: (1) change in level, (2) change in slope, and (3) the presence of drift.

Each phase should be compared in regards to level, slope, and drift. A change in level refers to the point where intervention is begun and baseline ends. A change in slope refers to a change in the linear directional trend between phases. Drift refers to whether or not a linear trend is present in any phase, and if the trend is the same across phases. This technique moves away from feeling or the experiential to a visual technique using models that are visually superimposed on graphed data. The models make use of the concepts of level and slope (see Figures 18 and 19).

Kazdin (1976) states that "a 'significant' change across phases will be reflected either as a change in level or change in slope or both." The following illustrations indicated a variety of possible experimental results. Each showed level and slope and interpretation of significances in terms of (a) no significance, (b) questionable significance, (c) probable significance, and (d) significance.

Here again, the importance of the interpretation depends on the client situation. For some clients, a change in level may be more important than the presence of a trend. For example, a change in the level of alcohol consumed might be indicative of a potential future change in slope; hopefully the slope will decrease. For other problems, levels might not be as important as the presence of a linear trend or a change in that trend.

It may be somewhat difficult to use this type of visual inspection on the raw data points if they are widely scattered, which is very common. "Raw" refers to the fact that the data points were graphed directly from the data collection schedule, and analysis was made from those original data points. The split-middle method of analysis does not alter those original data points, but rather summarizes the data points in a way that characterizes the data and can refine the visual inspection mode of analysis.

84

Figure 18.

ILLUSTRATIONS OF LEVEL, SLOPE, AND DRIFT*

A. Level

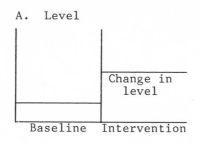

B. Slope or Trend

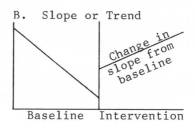

C. Drift (trend across or
    within phases)

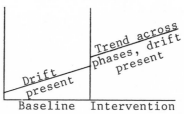

*All three concepts can be explored in example A, B,
or C. Only for the purposes of clarity and simplicity
have they been considered one at a time.

Figure 19.

ILLUSTRATIONS AND INTERPRETATIONS
OF A VISUAL INSPECTION METHOD

Rate of
weight
loss

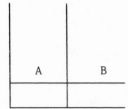

a. No change in
level or
slope. No
drift across
or within
phases.

Rate of
weight
loss

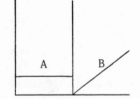

b. Change in
level but no
change in
slope. No
drift across
or within
phases.

Rate of
weight
loss

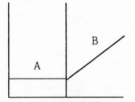

c. No change in
level, change
in slope.
Questionable
drift across
phases. Drift
present in
phase B.

Rate of
weight
loss

d. Change in
level and
slope. Drift
present in
phase B.

Rate of
weight
loss

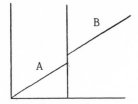

e. Change in
   level, no
   change in
   slope. Drift
   across and
   within phases.

Rate of
weight
loss

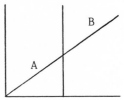

f. No change in
   level, no
   change in
   slope. Drift
   within and
   across phases.

Rate of
weight
loss

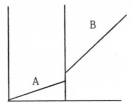

g. Change in level
   and slope.
   Probable drift
   within and
   across phases.

Rate of
weight
loss

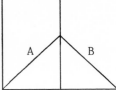

h. No change in
   level, change
   in slope.
   Drift present
   within each
   phase, not
   across phases
   since the
   drifts are in
   the opposite
   direction.

CHAPTER 7

STATISTICAL TECHNIQUES FOR DATA ANALYSIS

The Use of Statistics

The use of statistics in the analysis of single case data has been a moot point. Historically the use of statistics arose as a means for analyzing groups of cases and making population generalizations and inferences. Since the experimental single case methodology in clinical work arose due to the dissatisfaction of the group comparison approach, antipathy towards the use of statistics is expected.

However, some statistical methods which are appropriate for the analyzation of single case data can be beneficial to reinforce visual inspection, to clarify uncertainties, and to provide more precision. Statistical measures should never replace visual inspection; these measures should augment visual inspection.

Statistical evidence may or may not be clinically significant. The practitioner's theoretical stance and knowledge of the individual case should guide him or her in determining the effectiveness of a particular intervention or the improvement in a client's functioning. Statistical evidence is not a substitute nor does it carry more weight than clinical judgement. It should be utilized as additional information regarding the single case project. In some cases statistical evidence may reveal small yet important changes. In other cases, statistical significance may only be indicative of a start in the right direction for a client. In any case, the practitioner does not have to decide between one or the other.

There are, however, some issues regarding the use of statistics. Most statistical procedures assume that the baseline scores are normally distributed and that each score is independent. The normal distribution is a theoretical frequency distribution in which scores will be distributed around a mean value. For example, the average amount of rainfall is calculated each year. Through the gathering of data through many years, we know that rainfall will vary around a mean and thus we can predict what the rainfull will be for a season or month.

The mean represents the most typical score and thus the rest of the scores are considered deviations from the mean. The average amount of deviation from the mean is known as the standard deviation. If a distribution is normally distributed, then 68% of the scores will lie within ±1 standard deviation and 95% of the scores will lie within ±2 standard deviations from the mean. Figure 26 is the familiar normal bell-shaped distribution. Most statistics are based upon these properties of the normal curve. However, use of the curve implies that the scores for each distribution are independent.

For our purposes this means that we must assume that Monday's monitoring is completely independent of Tuesday's monitoring. In time series analysis, of which single case is a part, the observation of one data point may influence or predict another data point. To the extent that one observation is dependent upon another, the data are <u>autocorrelated</u>. Correlation is a common statistical procedure which measures covariation, or to what extent one event may predict another, although correlation does not by itself imply causation. Autocorrelation measures to what extent one event predicts the <u>same</u> event at a later time point. This problem for the most part is a mathematical property and usually cannot be detected by visual inspection. If the data are autocorrelated this may confound any statistical testing. Fortunately, there is a relatively easy computational method to check for autocorrelation or serial dependency. Some researchers suggest to test for autocorrelation before using any statistical procedures, and others suggest that the researcher be cognizant of the possibility of serial dependency and proceed as usual. If the data are not autocorrelated, then one can use the data as it is; however, if the data are serially dependent, then theoretically the data is to be transformed to remove the dependency.

The computational steps necessary to test for autocorrelation are presented in Bloom and Fisher (1982). Because the statistics used in single subject research are easy to conceptualize and calculate and yield very useful information, regardless of whether significance is attained, testing for autocorrelation may certainly be worth the few minutes it takes. On the other hand, not testing does not prohibit the use of the statistics which will be presented. One should exercise caution, however, in using them as hard, substantive evidence.

Figure 26.

THE NORMAL CURVE: Proportion of Area Falling Within Ordinates
at Specified Standard Deviation Units From the Mean

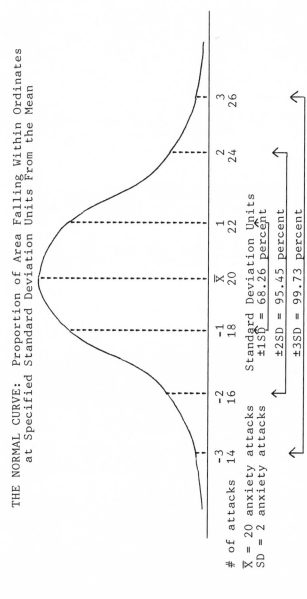

| # of attacks | -3
14 | -2
16 | -1
18 | $\overline{X}$
20 | 1
22 | 2
24 | 3
26 |

$\overline{X}$ = 20 anxiety attacks
SD = 2 anxiety attacks

Standard Deviation Units
±1SD = 68.26 percent
±2SD = 95.45 percent
±3SD = 99.73 percent

Illustration: For illustrative purposes let us assume that the target behavior being
monitored is the number of anxiety attacks (as defined by the client). If the baseline data are normally distributed, then 68% of the baseline data will be within one
standard deviation from the mean. Thus, this person had a range of 18 to 22 attacks
68% of the time, and we would know that from 14-26 attacks encompasses 95% of the
baseline data points.

If the data are autocorrelated one can use such methods as the Moving Averages approach (see Bloom and Fisher, 1982). The transformed data then is used in the statistical computations. Of course, one may still choose to use the original data even if the test for autocorrelation is significant to show exactly at what levels behavior or feelings were before and during intervention.

Statistical Significance

Both the celeration line and relative frequency approach, which will be discussed next, make use of probability tables. Probability can be defined as the ratio of:

$$\frac{\text{No. of Times a Specific Event Occurs}}{\text{Total No. of Events}}$$

Applied to single case designs, we may be interested in the number of times a desirable event occurred during baseline, and then during intervention. If the ratio during intervention is higher than that during base-line, can we infer that the change was due to the intervention? Obviously we would like to. For example, if the target behavior, assertive behavior, increased when the intervention of counting the number of utterances of the word "No" was applied, we would like to infer that the counting and consequent awareness was responsible for the increased assertive behavior. The fact remains that we will never be able to say with 100% certainty that it was the intervention. However, we could make a statistical statement that will provide us with a specified level of certainty.

How likely is it that the desired behavior increased as a result of the intervention, and not as a result of chance factors? This is a statistical question that is extremely relevant to the practitioner's purposes. By consulting a probability table, one can easily ascertain whether or not an increase or decrease in behavior or mood levels (depending on the measure and instrument) was significant. Significant denotes that the occurrence was not due to chance factors, but rather to something else.

The practitioner decides in each case what level of significance to assume. Does one want to say with 95% confidence that this result (a change from one phase to another) is significant? If so, one is assuming only a 5% risk of being wrong. In social scientific research the .05 level is most commonly used. If one would like to assume only a 1/100 risk of being wrong, a .01 significance level is assumed and if the result is significant, this would signify that this result is so rare that it couldn't possibly be due to chance factors. It would only be due to chance factors 1% of the time.

In single case research, then, we can look at the number of intervention events, and ask ourselves, is this a real change from baseline or withdrawal, or is the change so common that it would be expected under any circumstances? Given the baseline, one can determine how much change must occur during the intervention phases in order to consider the result a non-chance (or very low probability of being due to chance) occurrence. This is the crux of the reasoning behind the use of statistics in single case research.

Using Statistics with the Celeration Line

The first statistical approach we shall consider utilizes the split middle method described in Chapter 6. It is important to note that the potential of serial dependency is not a concern in using this method. Since the celeration line is a measure of the trend in the data, the problem of autocorrelation is already taken into account. In fact, Bloom and Fisher, in their text (1982), suggest that the celeration line technique may bridge the gap between the problem of autocorrelation and the use of statistics.

After the celeration line is drawn for the baseline phase, extend it into the next phase. Simply use a straight edge and project the celeration line into the next phase. The next step is to determine where desirable behavior is, either above or below the celeration line. Then, determine the proportion of baseline observations (data points) which fall above or below the celeration line. To do this, count the number of observations above or below the baseline celeration line and divide by the total number of baseline observations. If the celeration line divides the baseline data exactly in half, the proportion will be .50.

Our question is, given this proportion in baseline, what does the proportion have to be during inter-

Figure 27.

CELERATION LINE PROJECTED FROM
BASELINE INTO THE NEXT PHASE

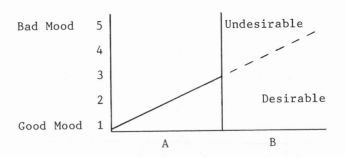

vention for a significant change to have taken place?
Are there enough data points above the projected celeration line to say there was significant change? To
locate just how many data points need to be above the
projected slope, one would consult a probability table.
These tables are very convenient to use, as all the
mathematical formulations have been taken care of.

One must first decide, based on the client situation and professional clinical what level of significance to assume, as there are probability tables for
various levels. In this text, we have included a por-
tion of the table derived for the 5% level or 95% confidence level. Of course the requirements for significance at the .01 level are more stringent, but the
levels of significance are not clinical standards, they
are probabilities, and have no inherent meaning in
themselves. In exploratory research, even a .10 level
of significance is often assumed.

To use the probability table, locate the proportion calculated earlier of baseline observations which
fall above the celeration line underneath and vertical
column labeled "Proportion" (see Table 5). If the
exact proportion is not labeled on the column, round
the proportion. The proportion should be around .50.

Next, along the horizontal row, locate the number
that corresponds to the number of days of the inter-

Table 5.

Table showing the number of observations of a specified type (e.g., a desired behavior) during the intervention period that are necessary to represent a significant increase at the .05 level over the proportion during the preintervention period.*

Proportion	Number											
	4	6	8	10	12	14	16	18	20	24	28	32
.05	2	2	3	3	3	3	3	4	4	4	4	5
.10	3	3	3	4	4	4	5	5	5	6	7	7
1/8	3	3	4	4	5	5	5	6	6	7	8	8
.15	3	3	4	4	5	5	6	6	7	8	8	9
1/6	3	4	4	5	5	6	6	7	7	8	9	10
.20	3	4	5	5	6	6	7	8	8	9	10	11
.25	4	4	5	6	7	7	8	9	9	11	12	13
.30	4	5	6	6	7	8	9	10	10	12	13	15
1/3	4	5	6	7	8	9	9	10	11	13	15	16
.35	4	5	6	7	8	9	10	11	12	13	15	17
3/8	4	5	6	7	8	9	10	11	12	14	16	18
.40	4	5	6	8	9	10	11	12	13	15	16	18
.45	4	6	7	8	9	10	11	13	14	16	18	20
.50		6	7	9	10	11	12	13	15	17	19	22
.55		6	8	9	10	12	13	14	16	18	21	23
.60		6	8	9	11	12	14	15	17	19	22	25

*Table of the Cumulative Binomial Probability Distribution--By the staff of the Harvard Computational Laboratory, Harvard University Press, 1955. Table constructed under the direction of Dr. James Norton, Jr., Indiana University-Purdue University at Indianapolis, 1973.

vention phase. The number on the table representing the intersection from moving horizontally from the proportion column and vertically from the number row is the number of data points needed during intervention to fall above or below (depending where desirable behavior would be) the celeration line for a change from baseline to intervention to be significant.

For example, if there are 10 days of the intervention phase and if the proportion of data points falling above the celeration line during baseline was

.40, at least eight data points during the intervention phase must fall above the celeration line, for any change to be significant.

The Relative Frequency procedure is very similar to the celeration approach as the probability tables are once again consulted to determine significance.

The Relative Frequency Procedure

The Relative Frequency procedure is based on the assumption that 2/3 of the baseline behavior represented by the data is the typical range of that behavior. To the extent that the data during treatment falls outside these parameters, significance is assumed, with the level of significance being determined by consulting a table of probability.

Instead of a celeration line being projected into the intervention phase, an area of "typical behavior" is projected onto the intervention phase. The proportion of behavior which fell outside the typical behavior zone (in a designated desirable behavior zone) during the baseline is calculated. And once again, this proportion is located on the probability table along with the number of intervention days to finally determine how many data points must fall outside the typical range and in the desirable range during intervention. Figure 28 is a guide to this procedure. And Table 6 below is a comparison and summary of the celeration and Relative Frequency approaches to data analysis.

We shall consider one more method in this chapter, and then review and summarize all three methods.

Table 6.

COMPARISON AND SUMMARY OF CELERATION LINE
AND RELATIVE FREQUENCY APPROACHES

Celeration Line	Relative Frequency
1. A celeration line (slope) is calculated from baseline data and extended into intervention phase.	1. A typical behavior zone is designated in the baseline and bands are extended into intervention phase.
2. Locate the proportion of data points above or below (determine if desirable area is above or below) the celeration line.	2. Locate the proportion of data points in desirable range zone.
3. Using a probability table, locate the intersection of the proportion and the number of intervention days.	3. Using a probability table, locate the intersection of the proportion and the number of intervention days.
4. Determine the number of data points which must fall above or below the celeration line in order to assume significance.	4. Determine the number of data points which must be in the desirable behavior zone in order to assume significance.

Figure 28.

RELATIVE FREQUENCY TECHNIQUE

Hypothetical Observations of Disruptive Behavior
Illustrating the Relative Frequency Procedure

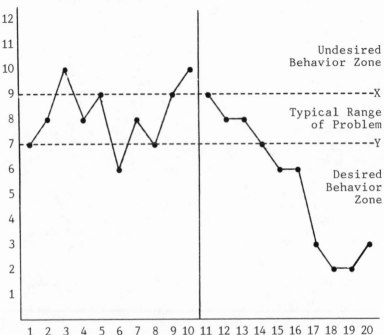

Guide to Computation of Relative Frequency Procedure

Step 1.   Count the number of observation points (score)
during the baseline period: There are 10
observation points during baseline.

Step 2.   Identify the typical range of the problem;
that is, the middle 2/3 of the baseline data,
by multiplying the number of observations by
2/3:

$$10 \times 2/3 = 6.7$$

98

Figure 28, continued

Step 3. Draw two bands to include the number of observations closest to the result obtained in
Step 2. At least one observation must be
above and at least one below the two bands:
Two bands are drawn to include 7 observation
points, the number closest to 6.7 with scores
of 7-9 being included. Two scores of 10 are
above the bands and a score of 6 is below the
bands.

Step 4. Calculate the proportion of the time a score
was found in the desired behavior zone during
the baseline period:

$$1/10 = .10$$

Step 5. Count the number of observation points (scores)
during treatment.

There are 20 observation points during the
treatment period.

Step 6. Consulting Table 5, in the top row find the
number of observations during treatment (10).
In the vertical proportion column find the
proportion of the time the target behavior
occurred in the desired behavior zone during
baseline (.10). Where the two intersect is
the number of observations that must be found
in the desired behavior zone during the
treatment period for the results to be considered significant.

According to Table 5, there must be at least
4 points in the desired behavior zone during
treatment. There are 6 such points in Figure
28; therefore, the results are considered
significant at the .05 level.

The Two Standard Deviation Procedure

The Two Standard Deviation procedure is similar to the Relative Frequency except that the desirable behavior zone is computed directly from the scores and not the number of observations. The two standard deviation procedure does not rely on a table to check for significance. It does assume a normal distribution and independence of observations, so checking for auto-correlation is suggested. If any two successive data points during intervention are located in the projected desirable behavior range, then the data in each phase are significantly different from each other.

Instead of assuming that 2/3 of the behavior during baseline represents the typical behavior of a person, use of this procedure assumes that the mean of the scores during baseline represents the typical behavior. Mathematically, remember that the mean, or arithmetic average, is computed from an entire set of scores; in other words, the mean takes into account every single score. One can think of the mean as a balancing point in a distribution of scores. The important property of the mean is that if one subtracts each score in a distribution from the mean, and then adds up each of these numbers, they will always sum to zero. This will not occur with any other number except the mean. Please refer to Figure 29 for an illustration.

Figure 29.

PROPERTIES OF THE MEAN

Data Points		Deviations from Mean Sum to Zero
x_1 3	$15 \div 5 = 3$	
	$\overline{x} = 3$	$3 - 3 = 0$
x_2 5		$5 - 3 = 2$
x_3 4		$4 - 3 = 1$
x_4 1	$\underline{1 \quad 2 \quad 3 \quad 4 \quad 5}$	$1 - 3 = -2$
	▲	$2 - 3 = -1$
x_5 $\underline{2}$	Balance	
$\Sigma x = 15$	Point	0

"Σ" means to ADD
"x" represents one data point

100

So if the data in Figure 29 represented baseline data of the number of cigarettes smoked each day, and if we wanted to make a statement as to the most typical amount usually smoked, our best estimate would be 3. Of course there are other measures of typicality, such central tendency measures as the middle score, or midpoint (used in determining a celeration line), and the most frequent score in distribution, the mode. All of these measures can be used when describing single case data; they should be computed for each phase. Thus by the mean baseline score, we have a summary measure that describes the average behavior or level during baseline.

After computing the average during baseline, the next question to ask is how much variability is there during baseline. In other words, by how much do the scores (data points) differ from the mean? Although the mean is useful, by itself it gives no indication of the variability. Were there very high scores during baseline which differed greatly from the mean? Or do all the data points cluster around the mean? Figure 30 illustrates the notion of variability. The mean could be the same for phase A and phase B, yet the differences from the mean could be very different.

Figure 30.

ILLUSTRATION OF VARIABILITY OF DATA POINTS

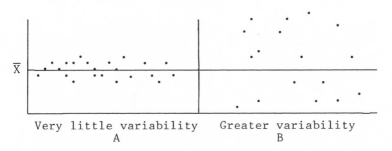

Very little variability   Greater variability
          A   B

In order to measure variability, the standard deviation is computed. This is a measure which indicates the average amount of distance each score is from the mean. Phase A in the previous illustration would have a smaller standard deviation than phase B.

The computational steps in computing the standard

deviation will be outlined further on. For now, let us discuss further the connection between the mean, standard deviation, and normal distribution in its application to single case data.

Baseline data represents the level of the target behavior and other dependent variables before any sort of intervention is applied. During this time, one is becoming more aware of the target behavior and its dimensions as they exist in the client's life. A mean of the baseline scores would theoretically represent a single measure of the typical level of the target behavior before intervention. However, as noted earlier, the mean will not yield information as to how and in what way the baseline scores are distributed. The standard deviation serves this purpose; depending on how the target behavior was measured (what is the range of the scale), one will be able to note not only visually by looking at the data points, but precisely the amount of variability.

If a distribution of scores follow the normal curve, then we know that 68% of all the baseline scores will lie one standard deviation on either side of the mean, and 95% of all the baseline scores will lie within two standard deviations from the mean, on either side. These are properties of the normal curve. Basically, this model is applicable to many events in life. With groups (many cases of individuals) we know that such physical characteristics as height and weight form normal distributions. It is not an absurd notion to apply this theory to events within one person. Most of human behavior is habitual and we can think of it having a mean level. Although we don't act and feel exactly the same each day, the variability would probably be distributed about a mean. Some days we may feel more or less happy, but we usually do not switch from ecstasy to mania. We do not think that manic-depressive symptoms are common, nor adaptive. Indeed, that person would have a very large standard deviation on a measure of happiness, while most of us would not vary so widely from the mean.

The Two Standard Deviation procedure, then, assumes that a typical behavior zone can be constructed by computing the baseline mean and standard deviation. By doubling the standard deviation, we have included 95% of the scores under the normality assumption. By drawing horizontal lines across the graph at two standard deviation points we can identify the typical range

102

of behavior for baseline.

Like the other two methods previously discussed, we can extend those bands into the intervention phase and see if any data points lie <u>outside</u> the bands and in the desirable direction.

Figure 31 provides a full illustration of this method and the computational steps. If two <u>successive</u> data points lie in a designated desirable behavior zone, outside the typical behavior zone bands, the intervention can be deemed statistically significant at the .05 level, which means you can say with 95% certainty that the data during intervention are different from baseline data and this difference is due to the intervention, and not to random, chance factors.

Figure 31.

TWO STANDARD DEVIATION TECHNIQUE

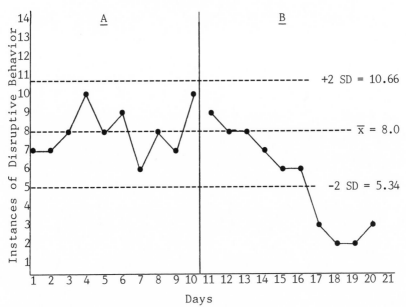

Change Over Time

Step 1: Sum baseline scores
Step 2: Square each baseline score and sum

103

Step 3: Square Step 1 value, and divide by N
Step 4: Subtract Step 3 result from Step 2 and divide by N-1
Step 5: Take square root of Step 4 value
Step 6: Calculate mean of baseline scores
Step 7: Determine 2 SD bands and extend
Step 8: If two successive observations occur below lower band, treatment is significant ($p < .05$)

Procedures

Step 1	Step 2	Step 3	Step 4
Day X	49	80	656
1 - 7	49	x80	-640
2 - 7	64	$(\Sigma x)^2 = 6400$	16/(n-1)
3 - 8	100		
4 - 10	64		
5 - 8	81	640.0	1.78
6 - 9	36	10⟌6400.0	9⟌16.0
7 - 6	64		
8 - 8	49		
9 - 7	+100		
10 - 10	$\Sigma x^2 = 656$		
$\Sigma x = 80$			

Step 5 (SD)	Step 6 ($\bar{x}$)	Step 7 (2SD)
1.33	8.0	8.0 + 2s or 2.66
$\sqrt{1.78}$	10⟌80.	[1.33 + 1.33]
		= 10.66
		8 - 2s or 2.66
		= 5.34

Summary of the Statistical Methods Presented

All three methods, Celeration Line, Relative Frequency, and Two Standard Deviation, are extremely easy to compute and are a very handy tool to assist in evaluating single case data.

All three methods summarize baseline data and pro-

ject what intervention could look like if typical behavior continued. The celeration line is a calculation
of the median rate of performance. The line is drawn
from baseline and extended into intervention. Since
50% of the data will fall above the celeration line
during baseline, if no significant change occurred,
then 50% of the data should fall above the celeration
line during intervention. The exact number of data
points needed the fall above the celeration line depends
on how many days of intervention there are, and with
this information, the probability tables can be used
directly. To the extent that more data points during
intervention fell above or below the celeration line
(depending on what was desirable) the intervention was
significant. One caution is to be exercised with this
approach. It cannot be used if the baseline data is
bounded. That is, if the celeration line reaches the
maximum or minimum during baseline, it obviously cannot be extended into intervention. The advantage of
this approach is that autocorrelation is automatically
taken care of. Another concern is to make both baseline and intervention phases approximately the same
number of days, since we are dealing with trend lines,
and time is a factor.

The Relative Frequency Method is less stringent
than the Two Standard Deviation Method in attaining
significance. For both of these approaches, autocorrelation is a concern. One does not need to consult
a probability table to use the Two Standard Deviation
procedure and it is highly recommended when there are
fewer number of baseline observations. Since the Relative Frequency procedure uses the number of observations as the basis for determining the typical behavior
zone, the fewer the observations, the more difficult it
becomes to use this method. Using the Two Standard
Deviation method is desirable here, since the typical
behavior zone is computed directly from the data and
not the number of observations. For both these methods,
a typical zone of behavior is determined and marked on
the graph. These bands are extended into the intervention phase and significance is determined by noting
the data points which fall in the desirable range.

Certainly these techniques will serve as aids to
make statements about the data, as to differences
between baseline and intervention phases. The practitioner may choose to use all or just one of these
methods, depending on the nature of the problem and the
type of data. This type of evidence may further rein-

force clinical judgements, or it may point to other noteworthy areas. Many practitioners using this method have noted changes in addition to the target behavior.

The methods presented here do not fully cover the range of possibilities. Other statistical analyses, such as a t-test for level, t-test for slope, analysis of variance, and various time series analysis models have been used (see Jayaratne, 1978). We have presented the most commonly used methods for practitioners. More elaborate and sophisticated analyses must be weighed in terms of their informational yield, and the ease in which they can be used, and the time which must be allotted. It is our belief that the methods presented here are practical to use and can fit within the hectic and complex schedule of the practitioner and client. This monograph was organized with that as a guide.

CHAPTER 8

COMPUTER APPLICATION

Introduction

Computer application refers to the storage and
analysis of data. One can use the computer for many
applications, including the analysis of single case
data. Computerizing the information (e.g., the data
collected from your study) involves transferring the
data from your data collection schedules to another
medium of storage, computer memory. Furthermore,
rather than hand tabulating and graphing, the computer
will produce means, summary statistics, graphs, and
charts electronically.

Why? Why would one want to use a computer for the
storage and analysis of single case data? Briefly, because of the precision and time gained, the flexibility
one could have in executing more elaborate designs, and
the possibility of accumulating single cases for nomothetic analysis.

It should be noted that the use of computers is
not essential nor even necessary for carrying out single
case designs. In fact, one of the advantages of the
method is that computers are not needed. But the point
remains that it can significantly enhance single case
studies. It is the purpose of this section to demonstrate how this can be done.

Furthermore, with the age of microcomputers upon
us, especially now in human service agencies, many
social workers may find that they have a computer available to them. In fact they may want to lobby for one
or be involved in the preparation for a computer system
in the agency.

What Is A Computer?

A computer system usually involves several parts
or stages. Basically, one can think of a computer system as an electronic storage device with mathematical
and logical capabilities. In other words, a computer
system can allow you to store information, and later
retrieve that information. The mathematical and logical capabilities built into a computer allow for all

kinds of transformations of data to produce statistics, graphs, tables, and various types of charts.

Most computer systems have an <u>input</u> device. The input device can be a keyboard attached to a terminal where you type information and see it displayed on a screen.

The <u>output</u> device is often a printer or maybe your screen again. Here you are providing a place for the results to be exhibited. In order to have graphs and tables produced a printer is needed. There are many different types of printers, including those which can produce graphs with brilliant colors or text with letters composed of millions of dots which form the letters.

Between the input and output devices are the computer's memory and the central processing unit (CPU). The memory comes in many sizes, stores the information, either temporarily or perhaps permanently, on disk or tape. The CPU is really the brain of the computer for it performs the mathematical and logical operations that it is instructed or "programmed" to do.

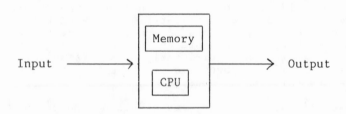

What has been described above is usually referred to as <u>computer hardware</u>. Also briefly mentioned above was <u>computer software</u>, or programs. Programs are the set of instructions needed for the system to operate. There are many different levels of programs from the basic internal ones that allow for the operation of the computer itself to the high level programs, or languages which the user gives the computer in order to produce a specific result. These high level programming languages are often known as <u>application packages</u>. The program itself is already written. All the user has to do is learn which instructions will give the desired result. The instructions most often are English sentence-like commands. These commands are recognized by the computer and then direct the computer to the program already written and stored in the computer. Some popular statistical application packages include SPSS (Statistical Packages for the Social Sciences) and SAS (Statistical Analysis System). There are literally thousands of computer programs which are used for word processing, accounting, spelling, statistics, data base management, and many other functions.

The type of program we would need is a statistical program or data base management system. In the future there may very well be programs called "Single Case Analysis Systems." However, there are many programs available which suit our purposes at least for the present.

Computerizing Your Data

Computerization is a synonym for the rapid movement and transformation of data. The movement first occurs from your data collection schedules to computer entry. Let us use Schedule 1 from page 58 in Chapter 4 as an example.

Schedule 1 includes nine items or variables. Each variable can be defined to the computer (via a program) and the values on each variable can be entered into the computer, again from within a program. Many programs are interactive, that is they prompt you for information after you begin.

After you enter the data from all the data collection schedules you would give the computer the program's instructions to tally each variable and produce statistics (means, medians, standard deviations) for each variable. You might want a graph of each variable by phase. With the graphs and the statistics, for example, the standard deviation, you could do the two standard deviation method of analysis in a few seconds.

GENERAL DATA PROCESSING PROCEDURES

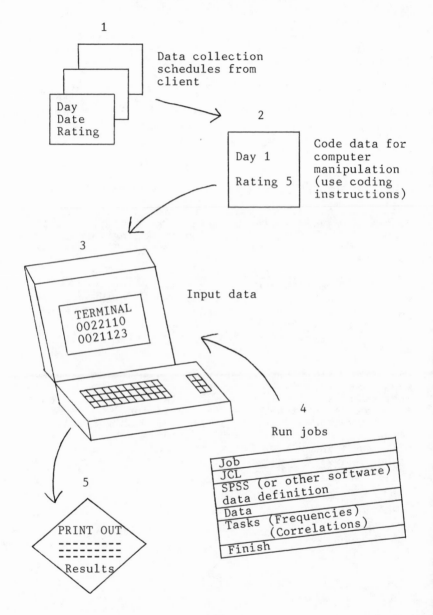

Discussion

One can go into great depth and technical detail in this type of exposition. However, we feel that the main point would be lost. That is, to consider the vast potential that lies in the application of computer technology to single subject designs.

Computers cannot do the interpretation of graphs and tables. That task will always remain in the hands of the researcher. However, the computer can greatly aid in this process.

The payoff for the investment in learning to use a computer, whether it be at the university or in your agency, is great. The computer can provide the most accurate statistics as well as prepare precise graphs based on your data. A large amount of your time is freed once the data are stored in a computer. You can produce multiple copies of charts and tables for drawing celeration lines or for marking in significant events. The multiple baseline or multiple treatment designs can be handled very easily with the aid of the computer.

Finally, though, we should like to end on a note of caution. To reiterate, the computer can save time and allow for more precision; however, it cannot replace the detailed interpretation that must be done. Furthermore, computer application should be not considered until all the methods of analysis are clearly understood and the researcher is able to do the analysis using manual techniques. It is difficult to think of a better way to learn these methods of analysis than by making your own graphs and computing the statistics using a calculator. Then it may be time to move to more sophisticated processing and analysis methods.

CHAPTER 9

A FINAL COMMENT

It has been suggested throughout this document that the use of single case methodology is not confined to clinical practice. Though the use of the method is still extremely limited in clinical practice, actual use of the method is applicable to a very wide range of problems and situations. For example, these writers' experience with teaching the method to undergraduates is marked by great enthusiasm and diligent application. Then, too, the range of problems is almost unlimited from medical, recreational, interpersonal to situational conflicts in the work or home setting. For the undergraduate it provides specific training and education in observation and differentiation of very subtle phenomena. It sharpens their awareness which feeds into their skills of interviewing and perceptions of client behavior which leads to effective diagnosis.

Clearly the applicability of this method of single case study to a wide range of issues and problems is not limited to highly trained researchers or human service professionals. That is, formal training is not required for effective use as evidenced in the frequent use of the method by clients in treatment programs. Of course, there are varying degrees of sophistication with which single case can be applied. In fact, the writers have always claimed that the basic elements of single case are already common to everyone's daily living experience. What we have strongly suggested is that these "common sense" practices be more systematically applied for more effective results and thereby providing sound evidence upon which appropriate action can be based. In effect what is suggested is the more general use of the method to produce human well-being as opposed to the exclusive use of the method by an elite group of professionals. Technology and in particular electric technology is breaking down the exclusive claim of the professions over specific technologies or "turf." This is clearly a positive move in the direction of democracy in health care, both physical and mental.

REFERENCES

Bloom, M., <u>The Paradox of Helping: Introduction to the Philosophy of Scientific Practice</u>. New York: Wiley, 1975. Chapter 17, "Worker Accountability: A Problem Oriented Evaluation Procedure."

Bloom, M. and Fisher, J., <u>Evaluating Practice: Guidelines for the Accountable Professional</u>. New Jersey: Prentice-Hall, 1982.

Boring, E. G., <u>A History of Experimental Psychology</u> (22nd ed.). New York: Appleton-Century Crofts, 1950.

Browning, R. M. and D. D. Stover, <u>Behavior Modification in Child Treatment: An Experimental and Clinical Approach</u>. Chicago: Aldine, 1971.

Campbell, D. T. and J. C. Stanley, <u>Experimental and Quasi-Experimental Designs for Research</u>. Chicago: Rand McNally, 1966.

Chassan, J. B., "Sochatic Models of the Single Case as the Basis of Clinical Research Design," <u>Behavioral Science</u>, 1961, <u>6</u>, 42-50.

Dukes, W. F., "N=1," <u>Psychological Bulletin</u>, 1965, <u>64</u>, 74-79.

Edgar, E. and F. Billingsley, "Believability when N=1," <u>Psychological Record</u>, 1974, <u>24</u>, 147-160.

Edington, E. S., "Statistical Inference from N=1 Experiments," <u>Journal of Psychology</u>, 1967, <u>65</u>, 195-199.

Gottman, J. M., "N-of-One and N-of-Two Research in Psychotherapy," <u>Psychological Bulletin</u>, 1973, <u>80</u>, 93-105.

Gottman, J. M. and S. R. Leiblum, <u>How to do Psychotherapy and How to Evaluate It: A Manual for Beginners</u>. New York: Holt, Rinehart and Winston, 1974.

Gingerich, W. J., "Procedures for Evaluating Clinical Practice," <u>Health and Social Work</u>, 1979, <u>4</u>, 105-130.

Hersen, M. and D. H. Barlow, <u>Single Case Experimental Designs: Strategies for Studying Behavior Change</u>. New York: Pergamon, 1976.

Howe, M. W., "Casework Self-Evaluation: A Single-Subject Approach," <u>Social Service Review</u>, 1974, <u>48</u>, 1-23.

Kazdin, A. E., <u>Behavior Modification in Applied Settings</u>. Homewood, Illinois: Dorsey, 1975. Chapter 4.

Jayaratne, S., "Analytic Procedures for Single-Subject Designs," <u>Social Work Research and Abstracts</u>, 1978, <u>14</u>, (3), 30-40.

Jayaratne, S. and Levy, R., <u>Empirical Clinical Practice</u>. New York: Columbia University Press, 1979.

Sidman, M., <u>Tactics of Scientific Research</u>. New York: Basic Books, 1960.

Thomas, E., "Uses of Research Methods in Interpersonal Practice," Polansky, N. A. (ed.), in <u>Social Work Research: Methods for the Helping Profession</u> (2nd ed.). Chicago: University of Chicago Press, 1975, 254-283.